Hidden Assets

Values and decision-making in the NHS

Hidden Assets

Values and decision-making in the NHS

Edited by Bill New and Julia Neuberger

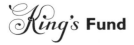

Published by
King's Fund Publishing
11–13 Cavendish Square
London W1G 0AN

© King's Fund 2002, except chapters 4 and 9

First published 2002

ISBN 1 85717 458 5

A CIP catalogue record for this book is available from the British Library

Available from:

King's Fund Bookshop
11–13 Cavendish Square
London
W1G 0AN

Tel: 020 7307 2591
Fax: 020 7307 2801

Printed and bound in Great Britain

Typeset by Peter Powell Origination & Print Limited

Contents

Contributors   vii

Introduction

Chapter 1   The values project   3
             Julia Neuberger

Chapter 2   Thinking about values   17
             Bill New

Thinking from the UK

Chapter 3   A Babel of voices: values, policy-making and the NHS   33
             Rudolf Klein

Chapter 4   The provision of health care: is the public sector   47
             ethically superior to the private sector?
             Julian Le Grand

Chapter 5   A tale of two tribes: the tension between   61
             managerial and professional values
             David J Hunter

Chapter 6   Democracy is king ... or mother knows best?   79
             Pamela Charlwood

Chapter 7   Values, ideology and the language of power   87
             Iona Heath

Chapter 8   Healing the multiple wounds: medicine   97
             in a multicultural society
             Ziauddin Sardar

Thinking from the USA

Chapter 9   Democratic decisions about health care: 111
             why be like NICE?
             Amy Gutmann and Dennis Thompson

Chapter 10   The trade-off between equity and choice: 129
              ensuring fair procedures
              Dan W Brock

Chapter 11   Managing disappointment in health care: 141
              three stories from the USA
              James E Sabin and Norman Daniels

Chapter 12   Caring for strangers: solidarity, diversity and the NHS   157
              Alan Wolfe and Jytte Klausen

              Practice from the King's Fund

Chapter 13   Voices, values and health: involving the   175
              public in moral decisions
              Kristina Staley

Chapter 14   Organisational values: a case study in the NHS   189
              Jane Keep and John McClenahan

              **A combination of thinking and practice
              from the UK and the USA**

Chapter 15   Refining and implementing the Tavistock   207
              principles for everybody in health care
              *Don Berwick, Frank Davidoff,
              Howard Hiatt and Richard Smith*

Commentary   The Tavistock principles: something more than rhetoric?   223
              Alan Williams

              Endword   227
              Julia Neuberger and Bill New

Contributors

Don Berwick
President, Institute for Healthcare Improvement, Boston, USA

Dan W Brock
Charles C Tillinghast, Jr University Professor of Philosophy and Biomedical Ethics; and Director of the Center for Biomedical Ethics at Brown University, USA

Pamela Charlwood
Chief Executive, Avon Health Authority, UK

Norman Daniels
Goldthwaite Professor, Department of Philosophy, Tufts University; and Professor of Medical Ethics, Department of Social Medicine, Tufts Medical School, USA

Frank Davidoff
Former editor, *Annals of Internal Medicine*, USA

Amy Gutmann
Laurance S Rockefeller University Professor of Politics and the University Center for Human Values at Princeton University; also Provost of Princeton University, USA

Iona Heath
General Practitioner, Kentish Town, London; and Chairman of the Committee on Medical Ethics, Royal College of General Practitioners, UK

Howard Hiatt
Professor of Medicine, Brigham and Women's Hospital, Boston, USA

David J Hunter
Professor of Health Policy and Management, University of Durham, UK

Jane Keep
Independent Organisational Development and Values Researcher and Consultant (janekeep1@aol.com), UK

Jytte Klausen
Associate Professor and Director of Graduate Studies, Department of Politics, Brandeis University, USA

Rudolf Klein
Visiting Professor at the London School of Economics and the London School of Hygiene; formerly Senior Associate at the King's Fund, UK

Julian Le Grand
Richard Titmuss Professor of Social Policy, London School of Economics; and Senior Associate at the King's Fund, UK

John McClenahan
Fellow in Leadership Development, King's Fund, UK

Julia Neuberger
Chief Executive, King's Fund, UK

Bill New
Independent Health Policy Analyst (bill.new@virgin.net), UK

James E Sabin
Clinical Professor of Psychiatry, Harvard Medical School; and Director, Ethics Program, Harvard Pilgrim Health Care, USA

Ziauddin Sardar
Writer, cultural critic and philosopher of science; Visiting Professor of Postcolonial Studies, Department of Arts Policy and Management, the City University, London; and editor of *Futures*, the monthly journal of policy, planning and futures studies, UK

Richard Smith
Editor, *BMJ*, London, UK

Kristina Staley
Freelance Researcher (kstaley@btinternet.com) and formerly Project Officer at the King's Fund, UK

Dennis Thompson
Alfred North Whitehead Professor of Political Philosophy and Director of the Center for Ethics and the Professions, Harvard University, USA

Alan Williams
Pseudo-retired Professor in the Centre for Health Economics at the University of York, UK

Alan Wolfe
Professor and Director of the Boisi Center for Religion and American Public Life, Boston College, USA

Introduction

Chapter 1

The values project

Julia Neuberger

At the NHS Confederation conference in July 2001, the Secretary of State for Health, Alan Milburn, made his usual speech to the assembled gathering from the NHS up and down the land. Towards the end, there was one surprising element, put in, no doubt, to reassure those who suspect wholesale handover of NHS services to the private sector in the light of leaks from various sources during the 2001 election campaign, and in view of a clear 'rule nothing out' view of what could be contracted to the private sector in recent private finance initiative deals. He said: 'We risk the ethos of the NHS, its values and its principles, at our peril. That is why we say, while we will forge a new relationship with the private sector, it is just that: a relationship, not a takeover. NHS values are not the same as private sector values.'[1]

So, what are these NHS values? And why should a Secretary of State, who clearly thought this talk of values was a bit 'soft' when he started in his role, have been persuaded to preface his NHS Plan[2] with a statement of values signed by the great and the good of the NHS and beyond, including the presidents of all the medical royal colleges? Why did talk of values suddenly strike a chord, and was this a genuine debate? Or was there something synthetic about it, something that allowed people to disagree about political principle without getting into the cut and thrust, and, as Rudolf Klein might argue, the precision of meaning, of political debate?

Certainly, in the mid-1990s, the debate seemed real enough, although the definition of 'values' was always fairly loose. The NHS had been through five reforms in the preceding decades and had seen its workforce become increasingly disorientated as new principles and values were thrust at them. There appeared to be a dissonance between personal values, organisational values, professional values, and a wider view of what the NHS was about, and what it was for. What had seemed to be a genuinely loved and valued institution in the UK for over 40 years, though always a political football, was now charged with impossible objectives and with competing values. Choice and efficiency, equity of access and effectiveness, universality and resource allocation/rationing according to ill-defined 'need', all appeared to have equal weight.

A group of us at the King's Fund decided to see if we could make any sense of any of this situation. We were helped by a US philosopher, Eric Meslin, who encouraged us to undertake an exercise in philosophical archaeology, looking at the stated values at around the time of the creation of the NHS. Although in the end the exercise was not as useful as we had hoped, it helped us see that there were three underlying principles at the foundation of the NHS: that it should be universal, comprehensive, and free at the point of use. Indeed, quotations from Nye Bevan exist which reveal that he was as attracted by the redistributive element of the NHS as by the universality of its provision.[3]

Although it is clear these three principles were the founding values, the 1976 Royal Commission on the NHS noted that: 'The absence of detailed and publicly declared principles and objectives for the NHS reflects to some degree the continuing political debate about the service.' So, we were not unique in thinking there was a problem. That problem, a lack of explicit values, was exacerbated as new values emerged. To universality, equity (of access and/or treatment), and free at the point of use were added effectiveness, efficiency, choice and user/consumer rights. The first two were adopted some time in the 1980s, under the Thatcher Governments. The last two came more slowly and almost more insidiously, and might be argued to be more important. They were not the product of political ethos in the same way the economists' view of effectiveness, efficiency and value for money was an expression of a world vision introduced by the Conservative Government of 1979. They came about as a result of a change in how people thought of themselves, a rising consumerism, a lack of respect for authority which had emerged in the 1960s and a gradual equalisation of the positions of professional and client. The NHS could no longer be as professionally led as it had been because users/patients now demanded choices, and the recognition that their views mattered. The all-powerful consultants were gradually losing out, in a revolution that was longer lasting, and far more important, than that which had brought effectiveness and efficiency into the list of values. Indeed, we are still seeing the power of the professionals decline and the gradual public awareness of doctors' fallibility has changed the way medicine will be thought of permanently. The doctors implicated in the scandals at Bristol, Alder Hey, and at Kent and Canterbury did not think of their patients as their equals.

So, things had changed significantly, and the revolution had been painful. The lack of confidence in doctors in the wake of various scandals was palpable and the public feeling that doctors said one thing but might well do another in practice, grew ever stronger, stoked by media reports of more and more 'bad doctors'. But this had to be set against what was already proving difficult – placing values such as efficiency and equity, against choice and consumer rights. As John Øvretveit wrote:[4]

> In many respects, choice and equity represent values held by two opposing political philosophies. Liberal and modern conservative ideologies emphasise individual freedom, responsibility and private property. Markets are proposed as a way of promoting these values and of advancing the common good ... Socialist ideologies hold that the individual realises their potential through collective action, and advance different forms of co-operative organisation and ownership as a way of upholding the interests of the individuals as part of society: equity and co-operation go together. The conflict between these two ideologies is greatest in the fields of health and social welfare, perhaps the last remaining sphere where the Marxist dictum is still widely held: 'from each according to his ability, to each according to his needs'.

Øvretveit is almost certainly right in believing that the tension between the two ideologies is most apparent in health. The fact that the NHS, with its origin in Beveridge's concept of the welfare state tackling the 'Five Giants',[5] was introduced in the immediate postwar period by a newly elected Labour Government, caused ideological tensions right from the start. Add to that the gradual distancing of the current Labour Government itself from the socialist ideal of 'to each according to his needs' because of a new concept of the Third Way and a realisation that consumerist societies in general, and the UK in particular, are less inclined to accept lower standards from public services than from private ones, and you have a recipe for confusion.

But that is not all. The values confusion does not lie only in the political ideology and the societal values surrounding the NHS. There are other value conflicts within, such as those shared by some of the professional groups who work in the NHS. Take, for instance, the doctors. They are not only adjusting to being seen as less than the all-powerful, utterly knowledgeable experts they were once considered, they also face a tension between whether they should consider the needs of each individual patient or the collective welfare of all their patients. Do they have a duty of care to patients, irrespective of cost in financial or time terms or, as primary care group or trust members, should they take into account the cost of treatments prescribed, and the cost to the practice of what is done for the individual? Will patients then think: 'Is he giving me this because he thinks it the best treatment possible for my condition, or is he giving me this because it is relatively inexpensive and will not make a huge dent in his drugs' budget?'

As we discussed these issues at the King's Fund in 1996, in an attempt to deal with them in a systematic way, it became clear that people from the professions and from the management side of the NHS *did* feel that their values were being compromised. This was in part because they often had to serve two or more masters, or because loyalties and accountabilities were somehow in conflict. Pam Charlwood, then as now, believed that purchasers of health care should promote dialogue about the values underpinning decision-making and that clinicians should play a wider role in the process, making explicit that they have to think both of the individual patient and about the good of the group. The tensions could be handled if everyone knew how the process worked, and that there was an explicit set of values governing decision-making. She and others, then and later, criticised the culture of assumed professional competence and superiority that would not allow for an expression of disagreement or acknowledge the need for trade-offs between different demands.

Equally compelling, back in 1996, was the heartfelt cry from Pam Charlwood and others present, for public service values to be recognised as a good in themselves. These are the values that motivate people to work for less money and fewer other rewards than they might receive in other sectors, in exchange for high esteem in society and a sense of self-worth. During this very early debate, the nature of the contract between the individual and society was raised several times. This led to questions about the desire to be beneficent (tying in with Beauchamp and Childress' four values for health professionals[6]), the value of health to an individual and the society of which he/she is part, and the value of care to the individual and to carers if a cure is not possible.

Once a set of values had been established that was broadly acceptable to those attending the first conference in 1996, the question of how philosophical the debate should be was considered. Should it be based on political theory? On formal ethics? And, if so, on medical ethics as established in the textbooks and increasingly in the professional codes, or a wider definition of ethics, such as situational ethics? Did we need proper philosophical training or could we manage with a loose form of debate, centring on situational ethics, organisational ethics and a series of values statements put up for debate?

And were we right in thinking that there were three underlying problems that needed to be tackled? First, the capacity of medical technology to treat far outstripping our capacity to think about the implications of that treatment. Second, the clash between the values and ethical codes of professional groups which focus on the patient–clinician relationship, and the values of the organisations where they work which require consideration of the group as well as the individual. Third, that the varying professional ethos and codes of the various players, including managers, needed to be pulled together to clarify that they had different goals and that trade-offs between value-sets had to be made. This would only be possible if the trade-offs were explicit – expensive treatment for the few versus far better treatment for the many; high-quality care without invasive treatment for the elderly, versus a sense that all that could be done should be done.

That first conference ended with a series of stories being told about where things had gone wrong and how being more explicit about values might have prevented the malaise often present in the NHS. From there, the idea emerged that a series of narratives might be useful to progress our work. These could illustrate where values were made explicit and where they were not, how organisations cope without explicit values, and where sniping within leads to a loss of confidence in the underlying – but not explicit – values of a hospital or other health care institution.

This was only the beginning. The debate took off, rather more enthusiastically than we had dared hope. Small groups began to meet to discuss values issues, culminating in a story-telling exercise and a conference where narratives illustrating values conflicts and trade-offs were acted out by professional actors. This became known as the Living Values project, an integral part of the early work on values by the King's Fund. Becky Malby and Stephen Pattison produced a report entitled *Living Values in the NHS – stories from the NHS's fiftieth year*,[7] which combined some of the emerging themes from that first part of the Living Values project. Marianne Talbot and Stephen Pattison both helped hugely all through its early stages in making people think clearly, even if most participants had had no formal philosophical training.

Marianne Talbot's emphasis throughout on organisational values was particularly helpful when health professionals from different disciplines, from doctors to managers, from nurses to estates staff, were debating what mattered within their organisations.[8] She also kept us on track when the discussion ranged too wide or when one or more of the participants took a purely relativist view about values – making them into personal preferences. It became clear that most people who engaged in the debate were nearer the position of Thomas Nagel, and his towering giant of a philosophical ancestor, Immanuel Kant, in believing that there was something objective and reasonable about values that people in a society, by use of their reason, could share. Marianne Talbot also helped organise a joint conference for health and education staff in early 2000 which explored the concept of a successful public service in a changing society.

Stephen Pattison, meanwhile, had made a particular study of the values of the managers,[9] demonstrating that they held a strong public service ethos, almost a 'faith', and believed they had the potential to exercise their power for the public good. Yet they felt overwhelmed by the often-contradictory policy goals which they were expected to endeavour to achieve. His work was lent even greater weight by the publication in 1999 of Jane Steele's report for the Public Management Foundation, *Wasted Values: harnessing the commitment of public managers*.[10] This made clear just how personally committed to making a difference public managers were, and how they held a public service ethos to be key to their thinking. Yet they often felt that their commitment was taken for granted, or even disregarded.

So, the Living Values project, which had started in 1998, but had its antecedents in the debate of 1996, grew into something bigger than itself. It became clear that looking merely at organisational and professional issues would not help open out the debate to the wider public. The decision was made expand the project, despite the misgivings of individuals such as Rudolf Klein, whose scepticism, beautifully argued, remains in his contribution to this volume. With the Institute for Public Policy Research, the King's Fund commissioned Bill New to work on the issue of trade-offs in values in the NHS. The resulting volume, *A Good-Enough Service: values, trade-offs and the NHS*,[11] began a wider debate, one which reached further into government and other areas. It recommended that the Department of Health or the NHS Executive should produce a statement of NHS values, but that this should be coupled with an explicit acceptance of the need to trade-off values against each other. To some extent, this recommendation has been accepted. The *NHS Plan* includes a list of values or principles at the front of the document, although there is no acknowledgement that values have to be traded-off against each other. The second recommendation was that government should lead a debate within this context, both about the nature of these values trade-offs and the possible development of decision-making frameworks to allow all those who work within and use the NHS to participate in their resolution. This has yet to happen, but a series of values seminars run by the King's Fund made it clear that there was real appetite for such a debate and the gradual evolution of local modernisation networks and boards may allow wider discussion of these issues. The third recommendation was that the education of all health care professionals should be updated so as 'to include the study of values and their conflicting nature; professional education needs to include a study of the NHS as a social institution with its attendant public goals'. This recommendation is also by no means fully recognised, let alone implemented, but some of the work on values described below may yet lead to a greater recognition of the need for change in the way health care professionals are educated in the ethics field and more widely.

From here on in it became clear that the Fund's work on values needed greater coherence. The King's Fund, as a keen advocate for opening up the debate on values, now needed to steer its own work. Under the leadership of Steve Manning, and with many other participants, we began to do just that. The work as a whole was designed to enable health care staff to give voice to their fears, hopes and concerns about the values of the NHS, and to learn to think in terms of conflicting values and trade-offs. Further objectives were to help to shape a real conversation about the values of the NHS, in particular, health, especially public health, health care in general, and then the public services more widely. Also, to encourage government and professional organisations to play their part in an increasingly urgent debate.

It was also important to involve NHS organisations which were keen to work on their values-based thinking. A values network was formed where they could work together, with facilitation from the King's Fund, on exploring their values more deeply, led by Judy Taylor. Meanwhile, work on public values around public health was undertaken,[12] commissioned by the Research and Development Directorate of the London NHS Executive. This was intended to inform the London health strategy in the new world of London governance, led by an elected mayor. This work, with the public being involved in making moral decisions, consistently demonstrated that Londoners favoured improving their collective health over all other values, which suggested a particular view about public good that was of enormous importance. Extrapolated to the NHS, it also suggests that the public is concerned about the good of the population as a whole, and does have a view about the shared value and values of its public health service. That thinking is explained in Kristina Staley's chapter in this volume, and gives credence to the view that the public is well able to have this debate, enjoy it, and engage with it, even though politicians often seem to fear asking people what they think.

Finally, a series of seminars was held, with a variety of speakers from the UK and abroad, to test out some of the key values issues, and to involve a variety of interested people in teasing out some of the questions with the speakers. What cannot be appreciated here is the enormous interest the seminar series generated, to the extent that those who wished to come had to choose one out of any three seminars, and places were at a premium. None of the organisers had expected such a response, but it convinced us that our timing was right – there was considerable interest, and identifying the issues for the wider debate was essential. This chapter concludes by focusing on this series of seminars and summarising the content of the resulting papers, some which are presented in this volume, though by no means all.

The first seminar was entitled 'Universalism and efficiency maximisation: the NHS – church or garage?'. Our speakers were Professor Rudolf Klein from the UK and Professor James Sabin, the co-director of the programme for ethics in managed care at Harvard Medical School and Harvard Pilgrim Healthcare. Jim Sabin has spent a considerable amount of time in the UK at various stages of his career, and is the author of the well-known and often-quoted *BMJ* article[13] about the differences between the NHS and US-style managed care. In the article he warns the British not to go too far down the managed care path. In this particular seminar, Rudolf Klein was sceptical about the whole values debate. As author of the original church or garage paper,[14] he predicated the whole debate on a search for a particular kind of 'decalogue' expressed in ill-thought through language, with a multiplicity of concepts, including principles, norms and objectives. However, he acknowledged that there was value in considering the eight 'values' that Bill New elucidated in *A Good-Enough Service*,[15] even if they were not all of equivalent importance or even of a similar nature. He also accepted that the conflicts between values – universalism versus efficiency, for instance – were worth expressing publicly and thinking through. He was much more sceptical about whether it was possible to draw any conclusions, or even whether, beyond expressing the conflicts, there was sufficient agreement about the precise meaning of these values to allow a debate to reach any useful conclusions or even political settlement. He also quoted something of huge importance, though people now tend to try to ignore or forget about it: Barbara Castle as Secretary of State for Health did indeed refer to the NHS as a kind of church: [15]

Intrinsically, the National Health Service is a church. It is the nearest thing to the embodiment of the Good Samaritan that we have in any aspect of our public policy. What would we say of a person who argued that he could only serve God properly if he had pay pews in his church?

Klein has described the NHS as a 'church for rationalists', created out of a missionary zeal born of the conviction that planning health care rationally and fairly was the best way to improve the nation's health.[17] In his description, Klein asked the question as to whether the NHS was still a church or now a garage, technocratic and efficient.

In a light-hearted editorial for the *BMJ* for its Christmas edition in 1999, I argued that it was still a church, in that it even now rests on a shared concept of collective responsibility, ostensibly therefore at least on a shared set of values.[18] Whether that can continue is an open question, and one that is explored in this volume by Alan Wolfe and Jytte Klausen in their analysis of a creeping change in ideas about solidarity.

In many ways, this analysis is the most challenging of all to a UK view of the world. What they suggest is that progressives in Europe and the USA pursued a politics of solidarity for a century up until the 1970s. That solidarity, leading to the welfare state, to redistribution, to subsidy if not provision of essential services, began to give way to politics with a new ideal – the promotion of diversity. 'The good society became one in which no person would have to live in shame because his or her gender, race, sexuality, or able-bodied status is different from the majority's.' They continue: 'Solidarity and diversity are both desirable objectives. Unfortunately, they can also conflict.' And, of course, they often do. This is one of the biggest trade-offs, where it is easier to feel solidarity with people who share your views, way of life, language, and so on. Yet, without a respect for diversity, social justice is hard to maintain. Wolfe and Klausen express one of the great conflicts in values in their chapter. Yet if we examine the strategic objectives of many organisations, including the King's Fund itself, the pursuit of equity (or social justice) sits alongside respect for diversity. The one might be seen, and has often been viewed, as a subset of the other. But the principle of solidarity, which came out of a sense of equity, can in fact easily conflict with the valuing of diversity.

Zia Sardar makes it clear that, if we really value diversity, then much of the value system underlying modern Western medicine needs to be challenged. Why is Chinese medicine described as 'complementary' when it is a system as solid as Western medicine? Why should one type of scientific view prevail? And why should the West claim the principle of free access to health care, when it began in the Abbasid Caliphate in 809AD? Sardar's words make a nonsense of some ideas about solidarity – precision in attribution becomes as important as understanding the trade-offs between diversity and solidarity.

So, although Klein is right to be sceptical, and equally correct in worrying about precision and meaning in the use of language, there are areas where conflicts are all too apparent. Equally, he is right to argue that we can only really judge people's values, and organisational values, when we examine the decisions they make and the actions they take. But the malaise that David Hunter points to in his chapter does have its roots, at least in part, in the 'absence of clarity of purpose in the NHS, coupled with various internal contradictions and conflicts'. Hunter continues that this sense of malaise and low morale in the Health Service 'may reflect a deeper problem, namely a lack of confidence about the NHS from within which inevitably fuels negative public perceptions of it externally'. But Hunter's view is that no progress in the values question can really be made without teasing out the complexities of a highly diverse and pluralistic health care system. And he proceeds to look at the tribalism in the NHS jungle, and to analyse the differences in attitude between managers and doctors, and the positions each group takes in the power play.

All of these arguments are essential, and Hunter's, in particular, makes it clear why the debate on its own will be of no avail. It has to be conducted alongside a far deeper examination of NHS organisations. This is why the work done by Becky Malby and Stephen Pattison was so important, and why the chapter in this volume about organisational values in the NHS by Jane Keep and John McClenahan deals so closely with organisational and professional/tribal issues. Our emphasis, all the time, on the question of trust was helped enormously by the contribution of Sir Cyril Chantler, Chairman of the Standards Committee of the General Medical Council.

Iona Heath's plea for a democratic function within the NHS is vital, tying in with Bill New's 'democracy' as one of the high-level values. Without it, users and providers cannot function with confidence. With democratic accountability, at least people know what is being offered, what they are entitled to, whom they are sharing with, and the nature of the political contract.

Heath's views on this are expanded in Pamela Charlwood's chapter. Charlwood sets democracy, one of New's eight values, in tension with other values. In particular, she makes the case that public opinion and experience are at odds with the views of appointed decision-makers or experts. Part of the difference may rest in belonging to different tribes – David Hunter's point in his chapter. But part is due to a real lack of public knowledge, which may mean poor disclosure on the part of authorities or experts. For example, the situation at Bristol Royal Infirmary, where various individuals and authorities knew that the success rate of the paediatric surgical heart team was far less good than other such teams, but told nobody. Or it can be less blameworthy, where authorities find something difficult to explain, such as where a concept is complicated, the science is difficult, and the analysis of risk difficult to absorb.

The area where the conflict really comes into play is highlighted by Charlwood's example of Bristol City Council's referendum to ask voters what they wanted to happen to their Council Tax. Pegging the Tax would mean a reduction in services, a modest increase would mean services remaining at their current level, and a larger increase would mean that improvements could be made. Forty per cent of those eligible to vote did so, with 53 per cent of them voting for the 'no increase–reduce services' option. The voters' preference led to reductions in services for children and older people, whilst a neighbouring local authority was less democratic, but services are being sustained. The question then is whether democracy in this case is 'right', or whether there are other values, such as equity, and protection of the weakest, of whom some cannot vote (children), where a paternalistic view might prevail. Or one could take the cynical view and suggest that the services, albeit well-meant, are not of real benefit to the weakest, and therefore there are other ways of thinking about all this. So, what is the lowest common denominator of unsympathetic 'vox pop' (and do we only describe it as such when we do not agree with their conclusions?), and what is true democracy? Are there ways of engaging the public to get a more considered, more generous, more community-based set of views?

Plainly there are other means of deciding on what matters, and what should, or should not, be funded. Amy Gutmann and Dennis Thompson's chapter analyses the National Institute for Clinical Excellence (NICE) as a decision-making body about drugs and services, from a US perspective. They come to the conclusion that ways of making controversial decisions have to spell out the legitimate public disagreements between valued ends and valued means and ends. They suggest a version of public discourse called 'deliberative democracy', which picks up on Pamela Charlwood's concern about the *vox pop* approach. They argue for this so passionately because it requires decision-makers to be open about the reasoning behind their decisions, as otherwise it cannot be debated. They suggest that NICE should also operate this principle, and give full and accessible explanations for its rulings, including, as necessary, cost and efficacy. There would still need to be trust in expert opinion, but, as they point out robustly, that does not imply blind trust. Professionals and experts would have earned that trust by a previous reputation for fair decision-making and by ensuring the process was made public and open to challenge. This approach goes some way to solving the inevitable conflict between democracy and other values such as equity and beneficence, where the experts are sure that they are doing good, but the public is not sure it understands or 'values' that good.

James Sabin and Norman Daniels, in their chapter on reasonableness in decision-making, take on some of the same concerns. They too look carefully at deliberation, and argue that listening alone will not do. They also argue that transparency is key to good decision-making, pointing out that the enraged response from much of the US public to managed care is because so many people felt the decision-making of the Health Maintenance Organisations was less than transparent and had more to do with cost than any other factor.

Dan Brock's chapter goes further and takes up the conflict between equity and choice. He argues that this problem is not exclusive to the UK and the NHS, explaining that in the health care reform proposals of the early Clinton administration in the USA, conflict was very much in evidence. The problem that lies at the heart of this conflict is that choice, by its very nature, might militate against equity, for instance, if many UK citizens decided to exit from the NHS and seek their treatment privately. Or if the rich in the USA simply bought up the best of the provision available. Choice suggests the capacity to get better, or different, treatment. Yet, in a system such as the NHS, the assumption is that everyone gets access to the same. If that were true, which it manifestly is not, then the choice would be between different treatments available 'on the NHS', or, and perhaps most irritating to health professionals, the choice of having no treatment at all. Though cheap in cost to the system, this is often very expensive in terms of mutual trust between professionals and patients, and suggests a degree of tension still between beneficence on the part of health professionals and autonomy on the part of patients and service users.

The final area of debate in this volume that touches an important arena in the broader discussion is that of public service. Julian Le Grand asks whether the provision of health care by the public sector is ethically superior to the private sector. If one takes the public sector as being ethically superior, that presupposes a view that altruistic motives govern those who work in the public sector, and that these are somehow intrinsically better than the motives of those who work in the private sector. That leads to a view that a system that relies on altruistic motives is likely to be better in quality and quantity terms than one that relies on providers motivated primarily by self-interest. Le Grand then proceeds to ask whether altruism can legitimately be separated from self-interest (there is a high degree of personal satisfaction in altruism), and secondly whether it is true that altruism is more prevalent under public sector provision than private. He then asks, even if it were true that altruism is 'better' and more prevalent in the public sector, if the private sector turned out to be superior in provision terms to the public sector, would it still be right to favour the public sector?

Le Grand goes on to show that there can be altruism and a public service ethos in private sector provision. However, he does not discuss what would happen if that very provision were largely funded, as opposed to provided, out of the private, rather than the public, purse. Is the public service ethos only to be found in the public sector, or can it be found in the private sector? And, if it can, does it rely on a fair amount of provision by the private sector on behalf of the state or is the nature of the ethos separate from the question of who pays?

Lastly, there are the Tavistock principles, discussed by Don Berwick and others. These were developed by a group of physicians on both sides of the Atlantic, trying to frame principles that apply whether the providers are public or private, owners of systems or deliverers of services through their employment. The principles are different from Bill New's eight, but are meant to be applicable in all kinds of health care systems the world over, and to go beyond the ethical codes of individual professionals, which can turn out to be divisive. What is interesting from a US point of view is that the Tavistock principles make health care a right, rather than something which one may or may not be wealthy enough to purchase. This resulted from the intervention of Amartya Sen, Nobel prize-winner for economics, who argued that by making health care a right, the debate had to begin about whose duty it was to provide it, and to ensure provision. This then gave an urgency to the implementation of principles which were fine in language but had little application in practice. Indeed, looking at them from a UK point of view, their impact would be limited. And yet a few organisations have experimented with using them in practice, thinking through their application in real time.

This volume encapsulates some of the main debates in the King's Fund series of values seminars. But it also goes much further. In pointing out where the conflicts lie, and where there are ways of resolving the conflicts by public deliberative debate and acknowledging value trade-offs, it leads us into a wider discussion of public service, public health, and, in the end, into the very nature of democracy itself. Can we have public services, provided by whomsoever, that can be clear about what they do and why they do it, and with a set of principles arrived at by reasoned, deliberative debate? From the limited evidence of the papers included in this volume, and the few attempts at deliberative democracy as yet undertaken, the conclusion must be that it is possible, though difficult. However, the process of thinking the issues through should lead to a greater satisfaction for NHS staff and for people who use the Health Service, because at least they will know what the Service stands for, and will have been involved in developing those principles into practice.

References

1   *Health Service Journal* 2001; 111 (5763): 11–12.
2   Secretary of State for Health. *The NHS Plan: a plan for investment; a plan for reform.* Cm 4818-I. London: Stationery Office, 2000.
3   The point is made in general terms in Timmins N. *The Five Giants.* 2nd edition. London: HarperCollins, 2001: 248.
4   Ovretveit J. Values in European health care markets: choice, equity and competition. *European Journal of Public Health* 1994; 4: 294–300.
5   Beveridge's Five Giants were: want, disease, ignorance, squalor and idleness, see: Timmins, 2001, above, p.24.
6   Beauchamp T L, Childress J F. *Principles of Biomedical Ethics.* Oxford: Oxford University Press, 1979; the four principles are: beneficence, non-maleficence, respect for autonomy and social justice.
7   Malby B, Pattison S. *Living Values in the NHS.* London: King's Fund, 1999.
8   Much of her work in this area was encapsulated in her book: Talbot M. *Make Your Mission Statement Work: how to identify and promote the values of your organisation.* Oxford: How To Books, 2000.
9   Pattison S. *The Faith of the Managers.* London: Cassell, 1997.
10 Steele J. *Wasted Values: harnessing the commitment of public managers.* London: Public Management Foundation, 1999.
11 New B. *A Good-Enough Service: values, trade-offs and the NHS.* London: Institute for Public Policy Research and King's Fund, 1999.
12 Staley K. *Voices, Values and Health: involving the public in moral decisions.* London: King's Fund, 2001; and in this volume, Chapter 13.
13 Sabin J. 'Mind the gap': reflections of an American health maintenance organisation doctor on the new NHS. *BMJ* 1992; 305: 514–16.
14 Klein R. The goals of health policy: church or garage? In: Harrison A, editor. *Health Care UK 1992/93.* London: King's Fund, 1993.
15 New B, 1999, above.
16 Cited in Klein R. *The New Politics of the NHS.* 4th ed. Harlow: Prentice Hall, 2000: 90.
17 Klein R, 1993, above.
18 Neuberger J. The NHS as a theological institution. *BMJ* 1999; 319: 1588–9.

Chapter 2

Thinking about values

Bill New

Oscar Wilde once famously described a cynic as someone who knows the price of everything and the value of nothing. This volume of essays is the result of a determined effort to avoid such a charge. Health policy over the last couple of decades has rightly been concerned with prices and costs; it is, whatever Oscar Wilde might imply, important to know the price of things because otherwise we cannot assess the implications of our actions. But perhaps too little attention has been focused on what precisely these actions are seeking to achieve. What are the objectives of the NHS and other public health care systems? What ethical principles guide the way we conduct public welfare services? What, in short, are our values? This book is devoted to an examination of the meaning of values in health care, their role and importance, how we might do better in applying and acting out values, and resolving conflicts between them. But before we delve into the substance of the issues themselves, we must first reflect on what is involved in thinking about values more generally.

'Value' is one of those words which at first appears easy to understand – it is in common usage, and even has a comforting familiarity. But on closer inspection it defies straightforward analysis and requires a rather extended introduction of its own. In this chapter I will attempt to set out as simply as possible the conceptual terrain which accompanies any discussion of values.[1] The first section reviews some of the semantic issues surrounding values; the second briefly discusses the competing views on where values come from; the third turns to an analysis of the difficulties encountered in producing and discussing a list of specific values; then, in the fourth part, I introduce the single most important philosophical challenge of thinking about values, and its implication for public services; finally, some key findings from this stream of work at the King's Fund are proposed. At various points I will refer to the chapters that follow, where some of these themes are taken up and developed in greater detail.

Moral and non-moral values

Our first clarificatory step must be to distinguish two basic types of 'value': the moral and the non-moral. Non-moral values are most common in market exchange. Consumers value products according to their tastes and preferences, and different bundles of products are associated with different levels of utility which, under conventional assumptions, the consumer tries to maximise. This process is understood to be a personal activity, with people simply assessing how much satisfaction or pleasure they are likely to derive from a good or service in the context of their endowed preferences. These 'values', tastes and preferences are usually taken by economists as given, beyond the reach of public policy,[2] and made irrespective of the views, tastes and opinions of others. As individuals we may not conceive of them as fixed in this way, but nevertheless we do not make economic valuations in the general expectation that others should follow our lead. Other people have their own tastes and valuations – strange though they often seem!

This personal form of valuation is also common in aesthetic judgements. Here, the medium will not necessarily be one of market exchange, but will usually involve a private assessment of worth. However, unlike purely market transactions, those who admire Mozart, Shakespeare or Jane Austen may feel that it is more than merely an expression of personal taste to say they value these artists more highly than Whitney Houston, Jeffrey Archer or watching *EastEnders*. They may believe there is scope for persuasion or enlightenment. Those who prefer the latter set may have formed their preferences in ignorance, or without proper guidance as to the qualities of the former set – although the 'uninitiated' will, of course, probably disagree. Nevertheless, these judgements are not normally considered to be moral, concerned with right and wrong, but simply the result of people having different tastes or, at most, of being more or less well informed or educated.

There may be other examples of non-moral values – such as whether to live an isolated, hermit-like existence or to develop human bonds of friendship and love. The latter choice is subject to strong pressures to conform in human society but, nevertheless, those who resist these pressures – who do not want to have friends or lovers, for example – are generally allowed to live as they choose. Indeed, such decisions are often rationalised precisely in terms of people holding different sets of values. In Western liberal democracies, at least, those activities which are perceived only to affect the individual undertaking them are generally respected, no matter how bizarre. Non-moral values, then, are typically distinguished by an understanding that people should be able to hold them in a personal way, unencumbered by the opinions of others.

Moral values, on the other hand, are concepts which are not purely a matter of personal preference. This is not to say that people cannot have different moral viewpoints, merely that when someone adopts a moral value position he or she will often be concerned if others adopt a different and opposing position. The key point is that values in this context concern assessments of goodness, desirability and rightness – to be contrasted with badness, undesirability and wrongness. People do not in general consider concepts such as these in isolation, with no consideration of what others think. Morality is a concept relating to how people ought to behave *generally*, even if individuals disagree about precisely what that moral behaviour should entail. For example, someone who opposes abortion cannot remain content if others carry out abortions, even when this does not affect them personally. The judgement that abortion is wrong (or right) is made not just with personal utility in mind, but with a more general understanding of what is good or bad about a certain form of activity. Sometimes this sensibility about the 'wider' good may act to constrain our own, rather more base and immediate, wants. So, the value of keeping promises may remind us not to go to the pub when we had given an assurance that the shopping would be done first.

But if we are not indifferent to others' moral values, it is at least possible in these examples for people to act out their different values simultaneously. That is, it is not conceptually incoherent for us to talk about people living side by side in society whilst holding diametrically opposed views on abortion. There are many other examples of this 'personal' form of moral value,[3] such as attitudes toward sexual preference, marital fidelity, using bad language, or religious conviction. One person acting out one moral viewpoint on these matters does not in practical terms prevent others from conducting themselves in a completely different way.

However, when we consider the activities of the state, it is not always possible for different value positions to be acted out simultaneously. In accordance with a key feature of public sector decision-making, public values involve collective decisions taken on behalf of a whole community. For example, if universalism is considered an important value in health care, then a decision might be taken to compel everyone in a community to be covered by a national health care system (no one can 'opt out' of the NHS in the UK). It will not be possible, however, for those who disagree with this value position to live out a different value – one which, say, involves freedom to choose whether or not to have health cover. If universalism is implemented, it must apply to everyone in the same way. The same applies to values such as equity or democracy – one cannot have more than one conception of these values operating at any one time for different people. Thus, 'public' moral values must be distinguished from 'personal' ones.

But we also need to define moral values more generally. Unfortunately, there is no consensus in the literature about precisely which definition best captures the subtleties involved. One attempt, taking a wider view than that implied by a focus on the NHS and public policy, defines values as 'qualities that are worthy of esteem …' and which 'generate' principles and standards.[4] An alternative approach emerges from an exhaustive review of attempts at definition specifically in the context of social science. Van Deth and Scarbrough distilled three elements common to most of these attempts:[5] values cannot be directly observed (they are ideas not 'things'); values engage moral considerations; values are conceptions of the desirable. We have already discussed the second two elements in the preceding passages; the first simply reminds us that values are not facts or empirical phenomena, even if we often attempt to elicit what people's values are by inference from their actions.

In the light of this it seems sensible to adopt the simplest and most parsimonious approach which incorporates the elements described. For our purposes, and in the context of the public sector, a summary definition is simply as follows:

values are conceptions of the morally desirable.

It is worth noting that although values are matters of morals, we might easily have said 'matters of ethics', and indeed we could have defined values as 'conceptions of the ethically desirable' with little impact on the sense intended. In everyday usage, 'moral' may imply censoriousness about personal behaviour, or religious strictures. 'Ethics', on the other hand, may imply an overly formal or academic concern, devoid of day-to-day relevance. Neither of these meanings is implied in anything that follows in this volume. In fact, in most philosophical discourse on matters of morals or ethics, no significant distinction is made between the two terms, especially when they are used adjectivally to describe a particular form of reasoning.[6]

A final point on definitional matters. Sometimes values can be instrumental, held because they lead to other more fundamental values, whereas on other occasions they can be intrinsic, held for their own sake – there is no 'deeper' value lurking behind. However, instrumental values are always subject to the empirical challenge of whether they do *in fact* lead to the more fundamental intrinsic value. Thus, instrumental values could be argued to be a quite different concept from intrinsic, which are not subject to empirical justification in the normal sense. For example, we might argue that maximising the improvement in an individual's health as efficiently as possible is intrinsically desirable. The particular mechanism by which we achieve that end is instrumentally valuable, and we might wish to test whether 'public service' systems relying partly on altruistic motivations are more or less successful than market mechanisms, such as the profit motive, in doing so. But matters can quickly become complicated when people start talking about 'altruism' and 'public service' as intrinsically valuable too. In other words, might we desire a public service system of health care, even if it did not produce as much health improvement for any given level of resource use than would a profit-motivated system?[7] Or is this simply a romantic attachment to the notion of altruism which, on closer reflection, cannot offer any intrinsic value beyond success in achieving health gain? For we would surely not support the incompetent doctor who offers her services free, over the brilliant but highly paid practitioner who achieves outstanding results – and yet there may still be something more agreeable about a system which is not dominated by personal gain. Perhaps such reflections make clear that many policy decisions require striking a balance rather than choosing between absolutes. A line needs to be drawn. Thinking systematically about values may not definitively draw that line, but it can demonstrate that policy options are rarely as straightforward as occasionally supposed.

Where do they come from?

Although we can all agree that values are not simple, observable facts – even in the way that people's statements *about* their values are facts – this still leaves a crucial issue in the debate about values and indeed their relevance to policy-making. Where do values come from? Do we have values as a kind of genetic endowment – like an emotional predisposition? Are they formed by our personal lifetime of experience? Or do they result from a rational analysis of issues, and thereby open themselves up to analytic refutation or proof?

In fact, these questions – about the origin and status of values – constitutes one of the longest running debates in moral philosophy, with two camps in direct opposition since the 18th century.[8] On one side are those who believe that values do not derive from reason but are essentially special sorts of 'emotions' or feelings, and thus differ between people just as other feelings and emotions do. We will characterise this group as the subjectivists. The 'godfather' of this lineage of philosophers is David Hume, with modern protagonists ranging from A J Ayer and the logical positivists, to Wittgenstein and Sartre, to contemporary writers such as J L Mackie.

Set against this group are those who believe that there is some objective element in values and morality, some principles which are true by dint of rational analysis, and that reason has a central part to play in the formation of values. There is often the implication that some values are indeed universal, not least because of their basis in rationality. The towering presence in this group is Immanuel Kant, with his categorical imperative to act, in moral terms, 'only on that maxim which you can at the same time will to become a universal law'. He believed that this was the only reasoned conclusion possible on the question of moral actions, and that therefore reason was at the root of morality. Other supporters of the role of reason in moral thinking include, in the 19th century, Henry Sidgwick, and in the modern era, Thomas Nagel. We will refer to these as the objectivists.

Without entering into a complex philosophical debate, the nature of the problem from a policy perspective is as follows. If, on the one hand, reason does play a role, and there is some objective, universal aspect to values, then there may be little point in engaging in debate about them. Instead, what is required is to educate those who have not properly understood what these 'objective' values are; to show them, as it were, how their reasoning must lead them to this conclusion. On the other hand, if people's values are simply a species of their feelings, then the policy-maker will not have much of a role to play here either – any more than they would in changing people's preferences for the colour of their car. If people do not sign up to the values relevant to the NHS, then there is little that can be done. A value debate *per se* is difficult; the task, in a pro-NHS camp, would be simply to establish what constitutes NHS values and then set up the political barricades against those who do not share them.

We cannot hope to resolve 300 years of philosophical disagreement here. However, there may yet be room for intelligent debate about values. Take the universalist, objectivist camp first. Although they would argue that values, strictly speaking, are objective, they would presumably not claim that there cannot be legitimate disagreement about the ordering, interpretation and application of these values in various circumstances. Kant established his moral law – the categorical imperative – and then went on to draw substantive practical conclusions from it. Others might agree with his philosophical basis and yet disagree about the implications: there could be a reasoned debate about this. A debate about the ordering and application of values is still a debate about values.

But what of the subjectivists? They are less flexible on the possibility of reasoned debate about values. A J Ayer argued that we often engage in disputes which are regarded as questions of value, when in fact we are simply asserting different 'emotional' points of view. For logical positivists, the only basis for debate with someone who has a different moral position is not to argue that this person has the 'wrong' ethical feeling, but rather:[9]

> we attempt to show that he is mistaken about the facts of the case. We argue that he has misconceived the agent's motive; or that he has misjudged the effects of the action, or its probable effects in view of the agent's knowledge; or that he has failed to take into account the special circumstances in which the agent was placed … We do this in the hope that we have only to get our opponent to agree with us about the nature of the empirical facts for him to adopt the same moral attitude towards them as we do.

However, Ayer's emphasis on facts may paradoxically leave the door open for a reasoned debate about values issues, even if it would not properly count as a debate about values for the logical positivist. Much of the kind of debate he alludes to is not a bald discussion of, for example, data reliability, but a much more nuanced and abstract discourse about how we perceive the factual world. Thus, we have the notion of 'insight': a particularly persuasive form of argument which makes us think again about how we understand events and situations around us. A critically insightful proposition about the nature of the world may often seem like a value position when in fact it relates to the complex nature of our *perception* of empirical phenomena. For example, a disagreement about capital punishment may not be based on fundamental value differences, but on what we believe to be the empirical impact capital punishment has on society, including its pernicious (or otherwise) influence on human behaviour in general, and on the likelihood of executing innocent people. This is certainly a debate worth having. But, ultimately, whether we call this a debate about values seems less important than accepting that people will continue to disagree even under the best empirical understanding of the issues, and that the challenge is to live together and respect each others' views as we do so.

Specific values

In a recent review of values which have informed the policy-making of the NHS, elicited from official documents over time, the following eight were uncovered:[10]

- health
- universalism (compulsory cover, etc.)
- equity (social justice, fairness, a fair distribution of benefits, etc.)
- democracy (accountability, answerability, etc.)
- choice (autonomy, freedom, etc.)
- respect for human dignity (honesty, consideration, fair dealing, etc.)
- 'public service' (public service ethos, altruism, non-commercial motives, etc.)
- efficiency (cost-effectiveness, maximisation, waste avoidance, etc.).

Now the intention here is not to defend this particular list but to suggest three sets of difficulties with producing any such catalogue of values.[11] The first relates to the fact that, as abstract concepts, many of the words which are used to signify a particular value have numerous close cousins, some of which may be synonymous, but others which have subtly different connotations with particular importance for different people. For example, Roget's *Thesaurus* gives the following alternatives for 'fair' (in addition to those noted in the list above for 'equity'): righteous, disinterested, unprejudiced, unbiased, detached, impersonal, dispassionate, objective, open-minded, egalitarian, impartial, legitimate; there are many others. Clearly, then, values related to being fair can be described in a huge variety of ways, leaving a bewildering array of terms and endless opportunity for semantic confusion and apparent lack of consensus. Examples are given in brackets of terms associated, closely or otherwise, with the remaining values in the list.[12] No single word will pick up all the nuances which reflect what is important in the concept for everyone, and thus a definitive list will always be somewhat unsatisfactory. There seems no alternative than to take time and care over defining values, and to avoid presuming that others will know what we mean when we talk about them.

The second difficulty is again linked to the problem of gaining a common currency for debate, namely, that it would be possible to have a shorter or longer list depending on how some of these individual concepts are precisely defined. In other words, equity could be defined very broadly to include concepts of personal dignity and universalism if one wanted to think of these latter concepts in terms of 'distributions' – everyone receiving equal respect and health 'cover', for example. On the other hand, one could separate out these concepts to emphasise what is particular about each, such as 'personal dignity' reflecting the importance of *relationships* between individual givers and receivers of care, and 'universalism' emphasising the *compulsory* nature of health cover governed by such a value. The reader will probably have his or her own idea about how the list could be rationalised into a different number of 'core' values. But it is worth bearing in mind that if we do design a shorter list we need to be careful not to disguise conceptually separate values. As we shall see later, these values can conflict with one another and we should not delude ourselves about the difficulties this can cause by failing to make such conflicts explicit. Of course, too long a list would be unmanageable, and so some degree of summarising is inevitable, along with a loss of subtlety and detail. We cannot achieve perfection in thinking about values.

A corollary of this need to summarise and simplify involves a third set of difficulties. In addition to there being a large number of semantic 'cousins', values exist in hierarchies. That is, 'high-level' values tend to have sub-sets of 'lower-level' values, which in turn have their own subsets. This relates to the increasing detail we may uncover when concentrating on a specific value: a 'desimplification' process. For example, there are many different types of equity – not synonyms for the word, but more specific types relating to different conceptual positions on what *exactly* equity should entail in practice. People who agree strongly that equity is highly important could differ markedly about which specific form should be applied. Thus, some might propose a strict concept of equal health improvement for all; others might argue for equal resource use in relation to need; others might argue for equal resource use for marginal met need, and so.[13] Democracy is another value which is liable to a huge number of interpretations about how it should be applied in practice. What this means is that the shorter the list of core values – the more simplification and generalisation we engage in – the more likely we will be to obtain a degree of consensus about them. But this consensus may disguise sharp disagreements about application. Again, the only way to deal with this complexity is to be painstakingly careful about describing what we mean when we say we value equity, democracy, or any other abstract moral concept, and not to ignore differences of value position by hiding behind generalisations.

Value conflict

I have suggested that public values constitute conceptions of the morally desirable. It might be thought, therefore, that even if definitions and precise meanings prove elusive, at least we should be able happily to pursue these values once we have pinned down their 'true' characteristics. But unfortunately the most significant values issue of all remains – indeed, it is one of the most significant issues of public life. The problem can be stated most simply as follows: many of the values we pursue simply cannot live together. Indeed, it is an unavoidable fact of human existence that the good things we desire are not obtainable without compromising our ability to obtain other good things. This applies most obviously in our consumption of private goods and services: with a limited income (and even the super rich have a limited income) we cannot consume everything we want. We have to make choices and trade-offs between all the valuable things we enjoy. Even those who can afford most goods have only limited time in which to consume them – choices cannot be avoided.

It is perhaps less obvious, but exactly the same process occurs when we consider values. Thus, at the personal level, values relating to family life, love and meaningful relationships may come into conflict with those relating to a satisfying and successful career. The pregnant woman may find her value for motherhood and the life of an unborn child comes into conflict with her own life's possibilities. Or the son who has to choose between honesty in informing his elderly, terminally ill mother that he, too, is terminally ill, or compassion for someone who 'need never know'.

Public values involve similar conflicts. At the most general level we may propose a number of 'high-level' or core values on which we can reasonably be said to all agree: equity, maximising the good, choice and universalism, for example. But it is clear that they do not always pull in the same direction. Maximising the total quantity of health produced by a community cannot co-exist with any particular distribution that its members might consider to be equitable; as we have noted above, choice does not happily sit in all its forms with a compulsory 'universalist' health care system; and democracy may throw up outcomes that conflict with any number of other values.[14]

Isaiah Berlin put it like this in the wider context of our to desire to promote liberty:[15]

> liberty is liberty, not equality, or fairness or justice or culture or human happiness or quiet conscience … If I curtail or lose my freedom … this may be compensated for by a gain in justice or in happiness or in peace, but the loss remains.

These conflicts are fundamental to human existence and are thus no less important to the conduct of public health care systems. The impossibility of combining some desired goals means, in effect, that achieving 'idealism' in public life – as elsewhere – is not just a practical impossibility but is logically incoherent. If we seek to achieve simultaneously all the values noted above we are doomed to fail. And yet the NHS is still described by its political masters as if it were immune from the normal constraints of earthly existence. It is, in Rudolf Klein's words, offered up as a church-like institution. People believe that, here at least, the normal compromises and imperfections of life can be avoided. Or that they *should* be avoided, if only politicians and others behaved in a decent way. But this is a delusion. And it is a dangerous one, because if the public's expectations of the NHS are continually failed, a diminution in political support may one day follow. Somehow we must leave this unhealthy form of idealism behind, whilst retaining the motivation to do good and act on the many values which idealism engenders.

Intellectual honesty and fair process

So, what to do? One conclusion is surely to develop a greater degree of intellectual honesty about the limits of public institutions to achieve all the objectives set for them. It should be a regular part of statements about the prospects of the NHS to admit and warn that it will inevitably 'fail' to achieve everything we value. For too long politicians have led the population to believe that all will be well if only they are given enough time to set right the ills of previous governments. But this is an immature politics; the ordinary user of the NHS may not have time to reflect on the subtleties of moral philosophy but he or she will listen and react to the utterances of politicians. Perhaps we are all ready to hear a message which is a little less extravagant in its promises, and which leads people to expect a little less from public services.

But even a greater degree of realism about the need to trade-off values and accept imperfection will not necessarily satisfy those who have to live with the consequences. Some people, as a result thousands of practical decisions made daily, will do relatively well, and some will feel they have been hard done by. The particular balance of value trade-offs at any point in time will not satisfy everyone. So, if one theme emerges from this collection of essays it is that attention must now focus on developing a fair *process* for making these decisions. The painful judgements involved in inevitably failing to satisfy everyone's desires must be undertaken in such a way that even those who come out with less than they believe they are entitled to, are willing to accept the decision. In the words of James Sabin and Norman Daniels, we need to do better in managing disappointment.

In five of the chapters collected here,[16] authors from both sides of the Atlantic suggest principles for guiding such decision-making processes. At the risk of grossly oversimplifying their proposals, I believe it is possible to summarise three key principles which run through them all: transparency, collaboration and revisability.

First, transparency demands that the thinking behind decisions should never be withheld from those whom it will affect, nor should the methods used to come to a particular decision. The practical and philosophical limits to what can be achieved should always be disclosed. And the reasons for coming to one decision rather than another should be openly expressed. Everyone should know who was party to a decision and what was said in the course of coming to it. There may be limits to openness but the general principle should be clear. Transparency also will allow the proper application of revisability – discussed below – because people will be able to challenge what they hear and see, but it will also cultivate a more mature climate in which the need for value trade-offs can be discussed.

Second, collaboration requires that those who are (potentially) affected by decisions should also be involved in making them, alongside the 'experts' and elected or appointed officials. The lay voice should be heard and included, in addition to the professionals'. This is not a call for power to be simplistically handed over to the people, but for the development of a genuine and continuous dialogue between those with the power to change lives and those whose lives will be changed. It will itself inevitably be a highly imperfect process – there are many more people potentially affected by a decision than can hope to be involved in its making – but nevertheless collaboration with at least some of the users of a service will inform and improve decision-making, as well as indicating to those who cannot be involved that accountability is functioning vigorously.

Third, revisability advises that all decision-making processes should be essentially humble. That is, it should be accepted that decisions will be made which turn out to be misguided or just plain wrong. Improved factual evidence may emerge, or an insight into the relative merits of competing positions will be presented which had not been considered previously. An individual may press his or her case successfully that some particular form of injustice has occurred as a result of an otherwise uncontroversial decision. In all these and other circumstances, the decision once made must be capable of being revised, probably by an independent body, and so the process must go on. Public policy must not deal in absolutes, just as service users must not expect miracles.

A transparent, collaborative and revisable decision-making process will probably have a greater chance of success in sustaining public support for institutions which must deal in collective decision-making – where individuals cannot hope simply to apply their own personal concept of the good. But such support must in turn must rest on a more mature understanding of the limits of welfare services such as the NHS, of their inevitable inability to live up to our most cherished ideals, and of their essential imperfections.

References

1   Much of this discussion is adapted from an earlier and more comprehensive discussion of values and their relevance to the NHS: see, New B. *A Good-Enough Service: values, trade-offs and the NHS*. London: Institute for Public Policy Research and the King's Fund, 1999.

2   Aaron H J, Mann T E, Taylor T, editors. *Values and Public Policy*. Washington, DC: The Brookings Institution, 1994. The authors argue that, on the contrary, public policy should consider its own potential impact on how people formulate their values.

3   Although we are not in general concerned in this book with values of this kind, Alan Wolfe and Jytte Klausen consider in Chapter 12 how different 'personal' moral values – deriving from different cultural and ethnic backgrounds – may affect support for public institutions such as the NHS.

4   Talbot M. *Making Your Mission Statement Effective: how to identify and promote the values of your organisation*. Oxford: How To Books, 2000.

5   van Deth J W, Scarbrough E. The concept of values. In: van Deth J W, Scarbrough E, editors. *The Impact of Value*. Oxford: Oxford University Press, 1995.

6   Furthermore, 'moral philosophy' is synonymous with 'ethics' in academic study. One exception to the similarity in usage is reported, but not endorsed, by Peter Singer in his Introduction to: Singer P, editor. *Ethics*. Oxford: Oxford University Press, 1994: 4–5; namely, that 'morals' refer to the customs and practices of different peoples in an anthropological sense, whereas 'ethics' refers to formal analytical study. See also Keep and McClenahan, Chapter 14 in this volume, for an example of an attempt to introduce a more significant semantic distinction between the two terms, and others.

7   See Chapter 4, where Julian Le Grand elaborates on this issue.

8   See Singer P, editor. *Ethics*. Oxford: Oxford University Press, 1994: 113–17.

9   Ayer A J. *Language, Truth and Logic*. London: Victor Gollancz, 1967.

10 New B, 1999, above.

11 See Rudolf Klein's chapter in this volume for an in-depth – and sceptical – review of this list of values.

12 'Health' is left out as this value presents particular problems; see New B. *Public Health and Public Values: resolving value conflicts*. London: King's Fund, 2000. Download from the King's Fund web site: www.kingsfund.org.uk/publichealth.

13 For a discussion of seven different types of equality, and an explanation of the relationship between 'marginal met need' and efficiency/maximisation, see Mooney G. Equity in health care: confronting the confusion. *Effective Health Care* 1983; 1 (4): 179–85.

14 Many chapters in this volume deal with these conflicts and trade-offs; see also New B, 1999, above, pp. 43–52.

15 Berlin I. Two concepts of liberty. In: Stewart R, editor. *Readings in Social and Political Philosophy*. Oxford: Oxford University Press, 1986: fn 5.

16 Chapters 6, 9, 10, 11 and 13.

Thinking from the UK

Chapter 3

A Babel of voices: values, policy-making and the NHS

Rudolf Klein

In a book devoted to exploring the role of 'values' in the NHS, it may be heresy to start a chapter by declaring a degree of scepticism about the current preoccupation with the concept itself. I recognise that our debates about the NHS are shaped by judgements about what is just or desirable. Nor would I deny that we tend to interpret 'facts' through the lenses of our preconceptions about what is just and desirable. My sense of unease has different roots. My contention is that the concept has turned out to be an extremely elastic one: that the process of exploring the notion has produced a proliferation of so-called values, a cacophony of claims about what the principles guiding policy and practice should be. The result, I would argue, is often to produce confusion, in particular about the relationship between ends and means and between seeing values as shaping policy as against being revealed in the process of making policy. Indeed, the word itself is in danger of losing meaning because it all too often is used indiscriminately and promiscuously: a sort of conceptual Gresham's law seems to be at work. In what follows, the reader should therefore imagine inverted commas every time the word appears.

In what follows I shall try to justify this claim. My strategy will be as follows. First, I shall address a puzzle: why the upsurge of interest in values – a fairly recent phenomenon? Second, I shall illustrate the confusion caused by the mass baptism of goals, principles and norms as values and question whether it makes sense to talk about NHS-specific values. Third, I will explore the ambiguity of many of the conventionally accepted values, and the conflicts between them, contending that they prompt questions rather than providing clear guidance. Lastly, I will argue that because of this ambiguity – and the fact that the signposts point in different directions – we only discover our values when taking decisions about what should be done. For all these reasons, I shall conclude, the quest for a set of explicit NHS values – a decalogue, as it were, to guide policy and conduct – may yield disappointing results.

Why the upsurge of interest?

The interest in values reflects the transition from seeing the NHS as a church to viewing it as a garage.[1] The NHS as created in 1948 was the offspring of a marriage between a moral imperative and technocratic rationality. On the one hand, the moral imperative was that a just society required health care to be made available to everyone: collective provision was the expression of a certain view of society. On the other hand, technocratic rationality seemed to require a health care system that could be planned purposefully and comprehensively in order to ensure that the wonders of medical science would be accessible to everyone. Morality, medical science and managerial rationality went hand in hand in what was, in effect, a declaration of societal faith in the ability of the new institution to deliver on its promises.

If the metaphor of the NHS as a church seems too far-fetched, consider this quotation from Barbara Castle[2] – one of Bevan's disciples and Secretary of State for Health in the 1970s – speaking at the time of a dispute over pay beds:

> *Intrinsically, the National Health Service is a church. It is the nearest thing to the embodiment of the Good Samaritan that we have in any aspect of our public policy. What would we say of a person who argued that he could only serve God properly if he had pay pews in his church?*

In other words, the NHS was seen to have both a moral as well as a scientific mission. It was not just saving bodies. It was also saving souls by embodying certain values of mutual help: very much the view taken by Richard Titmuss in *The Gift Relationship*,[3] his celebration of the NHS as an instrument for promoting a communitarian vision of society. The universality of the health care system was seen not just as the means of ensuring access to all, but as the celebration of the common humanity of all citizens: rich and poor are treated alike in the cancer ward.

Moving to the 1980s, there was a transformation – a process of secularisation – towards viewing the NHS as a garage instead of a church. Faith in the medical science was no longer as blind as in 1948. There was a linguistic revolution: the transformation of the patient into a consumer. The patient is someone to whom things are done. It implies a passive role. The consumer is someone who goes out to satisfy his or her wants, an active role. The emphasis switched from seeing the NHS as an instrument for promoting broad social goals, such as social cohesion, to seeing it as satisfying individual expectations: specifically, expectations that people will get an efficient repair and maintenance service (and will switch to a different garage if those expectations are not met – a rising trend in the 1980s, as the expansion of the private sector of health care demonstrated).

The change threatened to subvert one of the assumptions on which the NHS was founded. This was that equity required that health care should be distributed according to need: essentially a technocratic-paternalist concept. For who would define need – and distribute (or ration) scarce resources accordingly – if not doctors and managers? Once the patient had been transformed into a consumer – once it was recognised that citizens and users were capable of expressing their own preferences or demands – there clearly was a tension. If belief in the principle of equity remained high – as reflected in the continued high degree of support for the NHS in public opinion surveys[4] – it sat uncomfortably with the new emphasis on meeting individual expectations and promoting choice.

There were other tensions, too. The moral vision of the ecclesiastical model was centred on the notion of equality. The new secular or utilitarian model put the emphasis on the notion of maximising the output of health care. Moreover, there were other developments which challenged some of the traditional assumptions. Increasingly through the 1990s, evidence accumulated that the NHS was not one of the wonders of the world: that other types of health care systems, whose institutional and financial design was very different, could provide universal protection often to a higher standard if also more expensive. And there was, perhaps most important of all, a transformation in the prevailing public philosophy. The assumptive world which had shaped the NHS had largely disappeared. The notion that rationality necessarily rested on state planning had become discredited. The new language of discourse stressed incentives rather than altruism.[5] The Protestants of the New Right challenged Old Labour orthodoxy; intellectual ecumenism – as exemplified by the Third Way – became the order of the day. In summary, then, the simple faith on which the NHS originally rested has come under increasing challenge. Hence the search for some landmarks to steer by: enter values.

A linguistic tower of Babel?

Axiological ethics – the study of values – is a recognised if low profile branch of philosophy[6] with its own technical language. But in everyday usage there is a cacophony of terms used to describe the notions of the just and desirable that should guide public policy and personal conduct: principles, goals, norms, and so on. Verbal profligacy can all too easily lead to confusion. Is it really helpful to put under the same verbal umbrella of values notions about the desired end-states of policy and about the means for achieving them? So, for example, a trawl of discourse about NHS values in official documents has produced the following catalogue: health, universalism, equity, democracy, choice, respect for human dignity, public service and efficiency.[7] Do all eight of these belong to the same conceptual family? Surely not. For example, the notion of 'public service' is different in kind from 'democracy'. It refers to the behavioural norms which should govern those working in the NHS, whereas 'democracy' refers to institutional norms which should shape public business. Again, it could be argued that universalism and efficiency sit rather uneasily in the list. Universalism may or may not be necessary to achieve some of the other goals, such as equity. But is it desirable in its own right? And, contra some economists, it is difficult to see efficiency as a moral imperative.

The list of eight NHS values, distilled from the language of public discussion about the Service, is a useful starting point for analysis, and was intended to be just that. But inevitably they reflect the NHS's own history and culture. It may therefore be useful to take a step back and ask what the values of a just and desirable health care system should be: to identify values extrinsic to the NHS, against which its design and performance can be assessed, rather than accepting the way in which they happen to have been contingently embodied in the institution itself. The former course suggests that the NHS represents some sort of ideal: that its values (however imperfectly achieved in practice) should guide policy and action. The latter course allows us to ask questions about alternative designs and futures.

So, for example, we might conclude that it is not even necessary to invoke the language of values to justify the creation of a universal, comprehensive health care system.[8] Prudent citizens under the veil of ignorance, it might be argued, would want such a system in order to insure themselves against unpredictable risks of ill health. A collective system of insurance, in other words, is simply the most efficient way for individuals to protect themselves, given uncertainty about how risks will fall, and on whom, and information asymmetries.[9] Seen from this perspective, self-interest, rather than idealism, is the driving force. The role of the state – given this line of argument – is then primarily to prevent free-riding by individuals: i.e. to make insurance compulsory. No appeal to values is necessary (except perhaps insofar as the statement that the state should intervene to prevent free-riding is a value judgement).

Less radically, and probably more fruitfully, we can explore the arguments used to justify state action to ensure the availability of health care for all and to promote health, based on more general considerations about the characteristics of a just society. Here the starting point is usually the assumption that health, however defined, is a basic good required by all citizens if they are to act as autonomous human beings and to have the capability to develop their potential.[10] From this it follows that everyone should have an equal chance to obtain the medical help and care that will enable them to achieve their potential as human beings (although, given constitutional differences, end-states of health will inevitably vary). Health care, it must be stressed, is not the only such basic good: the list – varying by author – can also include political freedom, education and a minimum income.

Two values seem to be central in this line of reasoning: autonomy and equity. And if we want to avoid the proliferation of values that follows from adopting a strategy of cataloguing the over-generous way in which the concept is used in practice, these two by themselves probably provide the necessary, parsimonious foundation for any analysis of the characteristics of a just health care system. For most, though not all, of the other advertised values can be derived from this founding pair. So, for example, choice is surely implied by the principle of autonomy. For how can people act as autonomous human beings if they are denied choice? Indeed, identifying choice as one of the principles that should characterise *any* health care system is rather more convincing than deriving it from the NHS's own values: choice is significantly absent in the NHS – not surprisingly so, given that the Service is a paternalistic-technocratic creation in its origins. Similarly, does not the equity principle implies respect for human dignity: i.e. treating all people with equal respect? We may still be left with some orphan values. Democracy is a case in point but, as I suggest below, there are difficulties about putting this forward as an NHS value.

As we shall see in the next section, even parsimony does not necessarily lead to clarity: equity, in particular, is a principle capable of many interpretations. But before moving on to exploring the ambiguous nature of so many values – and the conflict between them – there is a further point which requires noting: i.e. that deriving a set of values extrinsic to the NHS – but which, it could be argued, should shape and inform policy and practice within the NHS – presents its own problems. If the NHS should embody or reflect certain wider societal values – such as 'democracy' – then once again we are faced with the difficulty of selecting them from a rather large, and not necessarily consensual, menu (even before we move on to considering just *how* such values apply to the NHS). Only consider the Third Way values, as expounded by Tony Blair: 'Our mission is to promote and reconcile the four values which are essential to a just society which maximises the freedom and potential of all our people – equal worth, opportunity for all, responsibility and community.'[11]

It may not be too difficult to translate some of these values into language appropriate for the particular circumstances and functions of a health care system. Some indeed echo the values derived from the arguments, already rehearsed, for establishing a universal health care system in the first place. Equal worth can be equated with equal respect; opportunity for all can be equated with the principle of giving everyone the chance to maximise their potentials, and so on. But the concept of 'community' – which appears to mean the promotion of the voluntary sector and initiatives by local communities – as a value in its own right introduces a new element. Should it be the function of a health care system to promote a healthy civic society as well as a healthy population? And how should we translate the concept of 'responsibility' into the context of the NHS or any health care system? Does it mean that the health care system should require citizens to accept more responsibility for their own health, and, if so, how?

All this, it may be said, is just academic quibbling. In practice, there seems to be general agreement about the principles that should be guiding the NHS: the eight values filleted out from the language of public documents and debate about health policy (see above). Since there appears to be a fair degree of consensus about these – cutting across political parties – why bother any further? The answer is that agreement about these values is more apparent than real. It rests on their ambiguity: the fact that they can be interpreted in many different ways. The next section therefore analyses some of the eight values in more detail.

Interpreting the oracle

Let us consider, first, the case of equity, a concept capable of many interpretations.[12,13] Here the conventional definition is that equal needs should be treated equally. But this begs the question of how need is defined and by whom. Should 'need' be defined exclusively by the professionals providing health care? This has been the traditional assumption in the NHS, which is precisely why I have described its dominant ethos as being technocratic-paternalistic. Or should the perceptions of those using the Health Service define 'need'? In which case, the definition of equity becomes equality in the ability to access the medical care which patients want. The antithesis is perhaps too neat. The definition may depend on circumstances. If I have a heart attack, and am lying semi-conscious on a trolley, I may well be content to have my 'needs' determined by professionals. However, if I suffer from a disabling problem with my hips, I may take a rather different view (and opt for the private sector, if I can afford it, should my definition of 'need' be different from that of NHS providers).

In defining 'need' in the NHS, professionals necessarily have to take account of the resources available to them: hence the much-discussed phenomenon of rationing. Should equity therefore be translated to mean using the same criteria when allocating scarce resources to patients, irrespective of their resources, social class or ethnicity? But the complications do not stop there. Depending on the criteria chosen, different patients will benefit. One criterion is to allocate resources to those patients who are most likely to benefit from medical intervention. Another is to allocate resources to patients who are most seriously ill, but have a lesser capacity to benefit. It is not self-evident which of these two criteria is more equitable. Again, to take an example from Le Grand's discussion of equity, consider the case of a drunken driver who hits a pedestrian out for a walk. Both arrive in hospital critically ill. Should both be given the same priority for treatment?

The problems are compounded when we move from considering equity in terms of outcomes rather than inputs. It is often assumed that inequalities in health outcomes[14] can be equated with inequity. From this it is concluded that if equity is indeed the guiding principle or value of the NHS, then its role should be to reduce inequalities in health: that evidence of inequality represents a call for action. But this does not necessarily follow, for two very different reasons. On the one hand, if poor health is the consequence of an individual's choices – like my own habit of cigar smoking – then it is difficult to see that the outcome is inequitable (unless one takes the deterministic view that all such choices are socially conditioned, dismissing all notions of free will). Only if an individual's ill health results from factors beyond his or her control is the situation inequitable. On the other hand, even if inequalities can correctly be classified as inequities, it does not follow that it is the responsibility of a health care system to remedy them. Given general agreement that the causes of inequalities in ill health are rooted in socio-economic conditions, this is to impose an impossible task on the health care system: social engineering is well outside the competence and capacity of the medical profession – even public health professionals. Hence, the absurdity of using inequalities in population health as indicators for judging the performance of health authorities.

If equity is a problematic concept, democracy is even more so – particularly when used (often inappropriately, I shall argue) in the context of a health care system. To start with, democracy is essentially a political concept: it is used – descriptively and prescriptively – to categorise the way in which societies design their institutions of government. Democracy, as rule by the people, is to be distinguished (to return to Aristotle) from both ochlocracy and aristocracy, the rule respectively of the mob and an elite. Having said that, however, there remain competing definitions of what counts as a 'true' democracy.[15] Do only societies which give citizens a direct opportunity to participate in decision-making qualify? And how representative do elected governments have to be to justify the label of 'democratic'? Is the protection of minorities from majoritarian tyranny one of the necessary conditions? The questions multiply as we seek an adequate definition of democracy.

Obviously all this is irrelevant to the NHS. Indeed, in many (perhaps most) respects, the NHS is the antithesis of a democracy. If equity is the NHS's guiding value, and if equity means distributing resources according to need as defined by professionals, then clearly talking about rule by the people is a nonsense. Technocracy and democracy pull in opposite directions. Taking a somewhat different tack, however, it is possible to make out a case for democracy in a looser, but no less important, sense as a value relevant to the NHS. Instead of agonising about whether the NHS is or should be a democratic institution (which it emphatically is not and cannot be), or speculating about whether elected health authorities or citizens' juries might make the NHS more 'democratic' in some sense or other of that protean word, we can examine its place in a democratic society and the extent to which its practices are consistent with those of that society.[16] This approach requires listing the conditions necessary (though probably not sufficient) for a society to claim democratic status, apart from the system of choosing governments. Such a list might include accountability, protection against arbitrariness, freedom of speech, the rule of the law and the transparency of the decision-making and policy process: in other words, a particular style of conducting public business and a particular kind of relationship between governors and governed – with the former never taking the consent of the latter for granted. To the extent that the NHS conforms to these requirements, it could also be said to reflect democratic values. But note, once again, that these are not NHS values in the sense of being specific to, or generated by, the Service; rather they represent a set of external criteria against which the performance of the NHS (or, for that matter, any national social insurance system) can be assessed.

Similar points could be made about most of the other candidates for NHS values. But ambiguity apart, there is a further problem. This is that the various values do not march in harmony. Here we come to the much-discussed dilemma – most famously by Isaiah Berlin[17] – posed for policy and practice by the fact that values conflict. Some of the conflicts have already been touched on. The notion of equity is at odds with the notion of choice: a needs-based Health Service like the NHS cannot, at the same time, be a demand-led Service. Efficiency, in the sense of maximising the benefits to society as a whole – on a utilitarian calculus – may be in conflict with equity, seen as treating all patients alike: it may imply (to return to an earlier example) treating those with the best chance of recovery rather than those who are most desperately ill and so on. Rather than elaborating on these conflicts – which have been well documented elsewhere[18] – the next, concluding section explores the way in which these tensions work out in the decision-making process.

The process of discovery

Much of the discussion of values appears to be based on the assumption that, by identifying them, we can somehow provide reference points for action, whether at the level of policy-making in the NHS or in the day-to-day conduct of its operations. Explicitness will provide clarity: a set of benchmarks against which to judge how we should take decisions and behave ourselves. But, as already argued, this is an over-simple view: the signposts point in different directions. If our real problem is to resolve tensions – to determine what weight to give to individual values in specific circumstances – then a somewhat different approach may be more appropriate.

In discussing such an approach – in moving towards what might be called a 'realistic' theory of how values feature in the process of decision-making – the best starting point is a distinction made almost 40 years ago by Vickers.[19] The policy process, he argued, represents a dialogue between reality judgements and value judgements:

> *The relationship between judgment of fact and of value is close and mutual; for facts are relevant only in relation to some judgment of value and judgments of value are operative only in relation to some configuration of fact.*

To put it somewhat differently, decision-making does not just involve a trade-off between different values but also means looking at the implications and costs (reality judgements) of adopting a particular set of 'value weights'.

In effect, we discover the weight we attach to a particular 'value' in the course of evaluating a particular situation or course of action: essentially a consequentialist process. In what follows, I illustrate this point.

Consider the case of private practice in the UK. Much academic energy has been devoted to investigating whether the NHS distributes health care according to need, and the conclusion is that on the whole it does so despite some geographical inequalities in the availability of services. However, the same cannot be said of the health care system as a whole: access to the private sector depends on the ability to pay. So, clearly its existence violates the equity principle. And if equity were our only guiding principle, the private sector should be banned (as it is, in effect, in Canada) or at the very least compelled to adopt the same criteria for offering treatment as the NHS (as is the case in the Netherlands). However, if we value autonomy, then a different conclusion follows. The autonomy principle means giving individual citizens the opportunity to exercise choice and to express their own preferences. Which is precisely what the private sector, though not the NHS, allows them to do.

The fact that successive governments have continued to tolerate the private sector might be taken to mean that autonomy rather than equity is the dominant value in the UK. In the case of Conservative governments, this might indeed be the case. But the same cannot be said of Labour governments, which have always stressed the centrality of equity in the provision of health care. Why, then, has the private sector continued to flourish even under Labour administrations? Enter reality judgements. The calculation has always been that the political costs of banning or restricting the private sector would be excessive: that it would be seen and resented as an infringement of liberty (all the more so since the same logic might seem to apply to private schools). Add to that the fact that it would also carry economic costs – expanding the facilities of the NHS and compensating doctors for the income lost as a result of depriving them of their income from private practice – and it is not surprising that inaction has been the norm. If Labour Secretaries of Health have any doubts about the political consequences of trying to give priority to the equity principle, they need only consult the history books: when Barbara Castle tried in the 1970s to implement her vision of the NHS as a church dedicated to the gospel of equity (see the quotation above) by limiting the scope of private practice, she was forced into a humiliating compromise by the medical profession.

Next, consider a characteristic of the NHS which makes it unique among the health care systems of the advanced industrialised countries: the fact that it is a centralised *national* service. Thus, it can be seen as a monument to the principle of equity, designed to ensure that everyone has access to the same package of health care, wherever they might happen to live (an ideal which, however, remains to be achieved). Further, it can be seen as a monument to the values of efficiency, the assumption being that a centralised service is a necessary condition for technocratic rationality. But it also seems to represent a repudiation of the democratic principle, insofar as 'democracy' can be equated with control by locally elected bodies. As Herbert Morrison pointed out in a 1945 Cabinet paper[20] – with resonance even today – criticising Aneurin Bevan's plans:

> *It is possible to argue that almost every local government function, taken by itself, could be administered more efficiently in the technical sense under a national system, but if we wish local government to thrive as a school of political and democratic education – as well as a method of administration – we must consider the general effect on local government of each particular proposal. It would be disastrous if we allowed local government to languish by whittling away its most constructive and interesting functions.*

But this is not just an example of trade-offs between values, with the twins of equity and efficiency triumphing over democracy. The apparent antithesis between the values concerned depends on a reality judgement. In contrast to Britain, the Scandinavian countries appear to be able to reconcile all three values: their health systems are not conspicuously short on either equity or efficiency and yet are run by local government. What distinguishes Britain is the judgement that local government lacks the necessary administrative capacity: a self-reinforcing judgement inasmuch as Morrison's fears have been realised, and local government has indeed increasingly languished as its powers have been whittled away by successive governments of all parties.

Finally, to take an example of a rather different kind, consider the debate about NHS charges. In the course of the 2001 election campaign, the Prime Minister returned to a long-standing Labour theme when he declared: 'If you're paying for basic health care, you're in breach of fundamental principles of the health service … I don't believe as a matter of principle that the NHS should be charging.'[21] In this he was presumably invoking equity, the notion being that any system of payment was incompatible with distributing health care according to need. But, again, a reality judgement is involved: that charges, even with large-scale exemptions for those on low incomes, are a barrier to access. There is indeed some evidence – though it is less than overwhelming –

that this is so. But would the same be true if, as is quite conceivable, it were possible to design a smart card which would allow charges to be more finely tuned to the capacity to pay – and if the system were therefore more precisely comparable to the progressive income tax scale which helps to finance the NHS at present? In which case, the principle or value involved might be thought to have less force.

In summary, then, there is reason to be sceptical about the usefulness of trying to carve in stone a set of NHS values to guide policy and practice. In the first place, the values that should be guiding the NHS should be those which are general to society, rather than being specific to the Service or to health care. In the second place, values are friable, in the sense that we only discover their meaning to us in particular situations. Their meaning – and the weight we give to them – will only emerge in the course of controversy and deliberation. An appeal to values – ambiguous, contestable and conflicting as they are – marks the beginning of argument, not its conclusion.

References

1   What follows draws on Klein R. The goals of health policy: church or garage? In: Harrison A, editor. *Health Care UK 1992/93*. London: King's Fund, 1993.
2   Cited in Klein R. *The New Politics of the NHS*. 4th ed. Harlow: Prentice Hall, 2000: 90.
3   Titmuss R M. *The Gift Relationship*. London: George Allen & Unwin, 1970.
4   Mulligan J A, Judge K. Public opinion and the NHS. In: Harrison A, editor. *Health Care UK 1996/97*. London: King's Fund, 1997.
5   Le Grand J. Knights, knaves or pawns? Human behaviour and social policy. *Journal of Social Policy* 1997; 26: 149–69.
6   Honderich T, editor. *The Oxford Companion to Philosophy*. Oxford: OUP, 1995: 71.
7   New B. *A Good-Enough Service: values, trade-offs and the NHS*. London: IPPR and King's Fund, 1999. In what follows, I draw extensively on this invaluable analysis.
8   Marmor T R, Boyum D. Medical care and public policy: the benefits of asking fundamental questions. *Health Policy* 1999; 49: 27–43.
9   Barr N. *The Welfare State as Piggy Bank: information, risk, uncertainty and the role of the state*. Oxford: OUP, 2001.
10 Here I am conflating (and over-simplifying) a variety of complex arguments produced by many different theorists. For examples, see Weale A. *Political Theory and Social Policy*. London: Macmillan, 1983; or, more recently, Sen A. *Development as Freedom*. Oxford: OUP, 1999.
11 Blair T. *The Third Way: new politics for the new century*. London: Fabian Society, 1998.

12 Stone D. *Policy Paradox and Political Reason.* Boston: Scott, Foresman and Company, 1988.

13 Le Grand J. *Equity and Choice.* London: HarperCollins, 1991.

14 Acheson Sir R. (chairman). *Inequalities in Health: report.* London: The Stationery Office, 1998.

15 Weale A. *Democracy.* Basingstoke: Macmillan, 1999.

16 Klein R, New B. *Two Cheers? Reflections on the health of NHS democracy.* London: King's Fund, 1998.

17 Berlin I. The pursuit of the ideal. In: *The Crooked Timber of Humanity.* New York: Alfred A Knopf, 1991; see also Williams B. Conflicts of values. In: Ryan A, editor. *The Idea of Freedom: essays in honour of Isaiah Berlin.* Oxford: OUP, 1979.

18 See New B, 1999, above.

19 Vickers Sir G. *The Art of Judgment: a study of policy making.* London: Chapman & Hall, 1965: 40.

20 Cited in Klein R, 2000, above: p.14.

21 *The Independent* 2001; 24 May: 7.

Chapter 4

The provision of health care: is the public sector ethically superior to the private sector?

©Julian Le Grand

In the last British election campaign, the debate concerning the relationship between the National Health Service (NHS) and the private health care sector re-ignited. It was stimulated by the leak during the campaign of a draft version of the final report of the Commission on Public Private Partnerships, a commission (of which I was a member) set up by the Institute for Public Policy Research. The Report was finally published a month after the election, generating enormous media coverage and, especially from health policy analysts and commentators, some vituperative responses.[1]

Despite the sound and fury, the Commission's recommendations with respect to private health care and the NHS were relatively mild. It emphasised the importance of the distinction between the public finance and the public provision of public services, and pointed out that a commitment to the former did not imply a commitment to the latter. It was critical of the various ways in which the private sector was currently involved in publicly funded health service provision, especially through the Private Finance Initiative. It pointed out that there was little consistency in the way in which the NHS used the private sector to provide health care, with extensive involvement in nursing home and in mental health care, but with almost no role in the provision of acute clinical care. It argued for a more consistent approach, one that would include a removal of the ideological barriers to the use of the private sector for the provision of clinical services. Finally, it recommended some cautious experimentation with private sector provision, with any such experiments being carefully monitored and their results being properly evaluated.

The extraordinary reactions generated by the Report – especially the more hostile ones – arose in large part because the issues at stake were perceived to be not just technical ones of the 'what's best is what works' variety, but ones involving values and morality. However, the latter were not always made explicit, and hence were not properly explored. Here the debate followed many similar private versus public arguments, where value issues are fought out under the guise of a technical dispute concerning different kinds of market and state failure.

This chapter is an attempt to address some of these value concerns directly. It begins with an exposition of the arguments put forward concerning the public and private provision of health care on both sides, distinguishing between those dealing with questions of value and those addressing questions of fact. It then subjects those arguments where value concerns are more prominent to critical analysis. There is a brief concluding word.

Private versus public provision

To begin with, the arguments against public provision. It is often claimed that public providers of health care are inefficient and slow to adopt technological innovations. They are unresponsive to the needs and wants of patients, showing more concern for the welfare of those who work within them than those who use their services. They have little incentive to change, preferring to stay with long-established patterns of working, particularly if these are in the interests of the professionals or other workers concerned.

In contrast, as supporters of private provision would argue, private sector providers, anxious to maximise their profits, are keen to eliminate waste, to adopt new technologies and working practices, especially if they look like being profitable, and to please their customers in case they lose their business.

On the whole, value issues are not brought directly into these arguments, except in one important sense. This is that greater efficiency, innovation and responsiveness are considered to be good things for the promotion of social welfare. Therefore, they constitute appropriate criteria against which to judge different forms of health care organisation. On this level, the argument is entirely an instrumental one: that is, it is trying to establish whether public or private provision is the better instrument for achieving these desirable social ends.

The case against private provision has instrumental aspects too, but also has another, more intrinsic dimension. To see this, it is necessary to examine it in a little more detail. Fundamentally, it is based on a combination of value and empirical propositions. First, there is the value judgement that altruistic motivations are intrinsically superior in a moral sense to self-interested ones. It is judged morally better to work with the aim of trying to improve the lot of others than to work solely on behalf of yourself. Second, there is the empirical proposition that the principal motivation of the private sector is self-interest, while that of those who work in the public sector is altruistic.[2] In other words, unlike private providers whose aim is simply to maximise profits, public providers' aim is primarily to help the people they are serving. This is part of the so-called 'public service ethos'. Taken together, this combination of value and empirical judgements implies that private provision is morally inferior to public provision.

The third proposition builds on the first two. It asserts that altruistic actions are not only intrinsically morally superior, but, contrary to the pro-private sector instrumental arguments, they are also more likely than self-interested ones to lead to superior outcomes – especially in the field of health care. In particular, health care provided through a system that relies largely on altruistic actions – on the public service ethos – is likely to be greater in quantity and higher in quality than that provided by providers motivated primarily by self-interest.[3]

Richard Titmuss was one of the most influential exponents of this kind of proposition, and the arguments that refer to quantity and quality can be illustrated by reference to his famous analysis of blood donation in his last book *The Gift Relationship*.[4] Titmuss argued that, if a system that relied upon donors giving blood voluntarily were replaced – or even just supplemented – by one where blood donors were paid, as some economists had advocated,[5] the overall quantity supplied would be reduced, not increased as the economists had predicted. This would be because those previously volunteering their blood would feel their donation to be devalued; hence, they would be more reluctant to continue giving, and would reduce the amount they provided. Although this was not explicit in Titmuss's argument, the implication was that this reduction in supply would more than offset any increase in supply generated by the payment incentives and hence that the overall supply would be reduced.

But Titmuss went further and argued that, not only would the blood supplied under a system of financial incentives be inferior in terms of quantity, it would also be inferior in terms of quality. Under a paid system, the suppliers of blood have an incentive to conceal any aspects of their previous health history that might have led to their blood being unsuitable for transfusion purposes (such as contamination by hepatitis B or, currently, HIV); for otherwise they would not be able to get their payment. This is in stark contrast to the situation where blood is freely given, since there the principal motive of the donors was to help recipients; hence, the incentive would be to reveal any history of bad health in case the gift of blood turned out to harm, not to help. Hence, blood supplied through a system that relies on voluntary donation is likely to be of higher quality on average than blood supplied in a market.

How does all this translate to the more general private versus public provision debate? It implies that, if private providers are paid to provide health care in a system that previously largely supplied health care through public providers, both the quantity and quality of health care would decrease. Public providers would feel that their altruism – their commitment to the public service ethos – had been exploited. In consequence, they would be prepared only to offer fewer services than hitherto and quantity would be reduced. State purchasers, lacking the appropriate information or monitoring tools, would be unable to prevent private providers from reducing their costs by cutting corners in their provision where they could, thus also lowering quality.

Titmuss[6] extended his argument from blood to make a moral critique of market incentives and private provision in general, arguing that:

> the private market in blood, in profit-making hospitals, operating theatres, laboratories and in other sectors of social life limits the answers and narrows the choices for all men. It is the responsibility of the state ... to reduce or eliminate or control the forces of market coercions which place men in situations in which they have less freedom or little freedom to make moral choices and to behave altruistically if they so will (p.310).

In other words, private provision is both *intrinsically* and *instrumentally* inferior to methods of service delivery that rely upon altruistic or professional motivations, such as public provision. That is, they are intrinsically morally wrong in and of themselves because they lead to self-interested actions displacing altruistic ones. This reduces the number and type of moral acts. And, as a consequence of this, the health care provided will be less, and of lower quality. Hence, the argument goes, private provision has no place in the delivery of health care.

Discussion

There are many issues here, and I do not have the space to deal with them all. Instead, I concentrate on three sets of questions raised, particularly, by the case against private provision, the answers to which are critical to the arguments involved. First, is it logically possible to separate altruism from self-interest? If not, then is it possible to say that altruistic actions are indeed intrinsically morally superior to self-interested ones? Second, is it automatically true that altruism is more prevalent under public provision than under private? Is the public service ethos unique to the public sector? It is apparent that the assumption of public sector uniqueness is crucial for the anti-private provision case; for, if in fact the public sector does not have a monopoly on altruism or the public service ethos, then public provision is not necessarily superior to private provision, either intrinsically or instrumentally. Third, what if both of these propositions do hold up – altruistic motivations can be separated from selfish ones, and they are unique to the public sector – but empirical comparisons of performance actually favour the private sector? Suppose it turns out that, despite its 'immoral' motivational structure, private provision does in practice provide a better quantity and quality of health care than the public sector. Should policy nonetheless continue to rely on public provision because of its intrinsic moral superiority – despite its instrumental inferiority?

Does true altruism exist?

First, the intrinsic moral superiority of altruism over self-interest. This is a value judgement, and hence not subject to empirical verification. However, it could be challenged on logical grounds. In particular, the validity of any sustainable distinction between self-interest and altruism could be denied. If someone performs an altruistic act of their own free will, then presumably they are doing so because they want to: that is, it is in their self-interest to do so. Hence, even altruistic acts are products of self-interest. There is therefore no case for elevating them to a higher moral status than apparently more directly self-interested ones.

This line of thought has a well-established historical pedigree. Thomas Hobbes[7] argued that everyone was fundamentally selfish even when engaged in apparently charitable actions:

> No man giveth but with intention of Good to himselfe, because Gift is Voluntary; and, of all voluntary acts, the Object is to every man his own Good (p. 209).

Bernard Mandeville[8] agreed:

*the humblest Man alive must confess that the Reward of a Virtuous Action,
which is the Satisfaction that ensues upon it, consists in a certain Pleasure he
procures to himself by Contemplating his own Worth* (p. 92).

However, there is also a history of rebuttal. Another philosopher of the
Enlightenment, Joseph Butler,[9] acknowledged that:

*Every particular affection, even the love of our neighbour, is really our own
affection, as self-love ... According to this way of speaking, no creature
whatever can possibly act but merely from self-love ...*

But he went on to argue:

*But this is not the language of mankind ... There is ... a distinction between
the cool principle of self-love, or general desire for our happiness, as one part
of our nature, and one principle of action; and the particular affections
towards particular external objects, as another part of our nature and another
principle of action* (p. 122–3).

To amplify Butler's argument, there does seem to be a moral distinction
between, on the one hand, those acts designed to be of direct of direct benefit
to individuals' own material welfare, such as their own personal consumption
of material goods, and, on the other hand, those acts undertaken that benefit
others: that is, acts that do not directly increase the actor's own welfare but do
so only indirectly through their positive effect on others. The fact that both
kinds of act may be 'selfish', in the sense that they both generate satisfaction or
some other kind of positive feeling in the individual concerned, does not affect
the fact that one act can be judged morally superior to the other. Hence, the
value judgement that altruistic acts are intrinsically superior to self-interested
ones cannot be overturned successfully on these kinds of grounds.

It is important to note that this does not in and of itself establish that altruistic
acts are morally superior to self-interested ones in a more general sense.
It merely indicates that the motivation for an act is one of the factors which
need to be taken into account in arriving at the overall judgement. Other
factors would presumably include the empirical question as to which of the
acts concerned actually does the most good to the other person. An altruistic
act that has no impact on the welfare of the person who is the object of the
altruist's concern is not obviously superior to a self-interested act that, as a by-

product, dramatically improves that person's welfare. Intrinsic moral superiority does not necessarily mean overall moral superiority. This is a point to which we shall return.

The public service ethos

The second proposition was the empirical judgement that those who work in the private sector are motivated primarily by self-interest whereas those who work in the public sector are motivated primarily by altruism. The difficulty with this, as with many of the empirical statements with which we have to deal in this debate, is the lack of evidence concerning it – and the often-contradictory nature of such evidence as is available.

One study that supports the proposition comes from a recent survey of the values of public and private sector managers by Jane Steele of the Foundation for Public Management.[10] This involved in-depth interviews with 17 top managers from the public, private and non-profit sectors, followed by detailed telephone interviews with 400 more. The study found considerable evidence both that public service motivations existed in the public sector and that they were much more pronounced than in the private sector. Out of 16 possible personal goals, the most frequently named goal of public sector managers was to provide a service to the community, whereas this did not even appear among the top ten goals for private sector managers. In contrast, for private sector managers the two (equally) most important goals were improving the financial performance of the organisation and achieving organisational goals or targets. Of these, the first did not appear among the top ten goals for public sector mangers whereas the second appeared sixth. Moreover, these differences did not fade with age or experience: they were not a feature of only the older generations.

However, Steele's study did not compare the motivations of public and private sector in the same line of business. Jeremy Kendall has investigated the motivations of independent providers (private and voluntary) of residential care and domiciliary care for elderly people.[11] In 1997, he interviewed just over 50 providers of residential care, asking questions about their principal motives for being in business. Of these, the most widely cited motive was meeting the needs of elderly people (80 per cent private, 94 per cent voluntary), while an equally large proportion (88 per cent in both) cited either or both of two other altruistic motivations: a feeling of duty and responsibility to society as a whole, or similar feelings to a particular section of society. This compares with the numbers citing the more self-interested concerns of professional accomplishment (76 per cent private, 75 per cent voluntary), developing skills (64 per cent private, 72 per cent voluntary), a satisfactory level of personal income (60 per cent private, 53 per cent voluntary), independence and autonomy (55 per cent private, 12 per cent voluntary), and income or profit maximising (11 per cent private, none voluntary). It is of interest to note that it is only with the last two, least-cited motives, that really significant differences begin to emerge between the private and voluntary sectors.

In 1999, Kendall and colleagues asked similar questions of 56 independent providers of domiciliary care.[12] On this occasion, they were able to provide the priorities given to the different motivations, as well as the number citing them. Of the respondents, nearly half gave as their most important motivation the altruistic motives of meeting the needs of elderly people (29 per cent), duty/responsibility to society as a whole (11 per cent) and duty/responsibility to a particular section of society (9 per cent). In contrast, only 13 per cent gave financial motives priority, while the remainder concentrated on professional accomplishment and creative achievement (21 per cent), independence and autonomy (11 per cent) and developing expertise (5 per cent).

Peter Taylor-Gooby and colleagues investigated the motives of British dentists choosing to treat patients privately or through the NHS.[13] They found that dentists were led to leave the NHS because of both self-interested motives and altruistic ones. By going 'private', they wanted to have a higher income and to have more independence for their own personal benefit. However, an important motivating factor was that they also believed that by so doing they could give more time and attention to their patients, and hence provide a higher quality of care. As Taylor-Gooby and colleagues comment, the interpretation they gave for their patients' interests was heavily conditioned by their professional culture (emphasising restorative rather than preventive work, for instance); however, the fact remains that patients' interests was a significant factor in their decision.

It has to be said that this evidence that different kinds of providers expound altruistic motives as part of their reasons for doing the job they do, or for making the decisions they make, is not exactly conclusive. It would be more persuasive if there was evidence that, actually, some sacrifice was involved (as in fact there may be in some cases where they are earning less than they might otherwise get for their skills). Nonetheless, the evidence, such as it is, suggests that there is a combination of motives in both private and public sectors: that neither has a monopoly on altruism or on self-interest. Hence, we cannot say unambiguously, *a priori*, that the use of either sector will be morally superior or respond better or worse in terms of quality or quantity. So, the proposition that the public sector is automatically better, both in terms of intrinsic morality and in terms of its ability to achieve other ends such as health care of higher quality or quantity, cannot be sustained.

Intrinsic versus instrumental morality

However, suppose sustained empirical investigation did reveal that, in fact, there was indeed more of a public service ethos, or more altruism, among public service providers. Would this trump all other arguments on the issue of public versus private provision? What if other empirical investigations showed that, for instance, relying on voluntary donation of blood simply did not elicit a sufficient supply of blood for the NHS's needs (however much public exhortation or campaigning was undertaken by the relevant authorities), whereas paying for blood or blood products did manage to elicit a larger supply, one sufficient to meet the NHS's needs? More generally, what if the instrumental arguments concerning appropriate methods of provision point in a different direction from the intrinsic ones?

As we have seen, Titmuss tried to avoid this dilemma in the case of blood by asserting, in effect, that it would never arise: that both the intrinsic and the instrumental arguments favoured the altruistic provider. He supported this by reference to comparisons between the blood supply situation in the USA, replete with shortages and breakdowns in supply, and the UK, where all needs for blood transfusion purposes were – at that time – being satisfactorily met. Unfortunately, his evidence was time-specific: within a few years of *The Gift Relationship* being published, the NHS was having to import blood products, and the organisation was a shambles.[14] More generally, it is not unreasonable to suppose that financial incentives could always generate a greater supply of any product or service – if they were large enough. Payments of, say, £10,000 per litre of blood 'donated' would probably be sufficient to ensure that the NHS had more than enough blood to meet its needs (although, of course, the quality could not be guranteed).

Faced with this dilemma, the advocates of the public sector ethos could respond with another kind of argument: that, even if a large enough supply of a good or service could be guaranteed by the use of financial incentives, relying on altruistic supply would be cheaper. Paying £10,000 for every litre of the blood it used, for instance, would probably bankrupt the NHS; relying on altruistic donations releases resources that can be used elsewhere for patient care. Thus, the greater good is served by the use of altruistic providers.

However, this instrumental argument runs into another, more intrinsic moral concern: that of the danger of exploitation. The blood situation is one where people are giving for free a commodity that, had they been less altruistic, they could have charged for (assuming that they were in a system that permitted the sale of blood). This parallels the situation of medical professionals where, it is often argued, because of their commitment to public service, they are paid less than they would have had to be paid if they were more self-interested. Is it morally correct to pay people less to provide a service than they would have received if they had been less altruistic? It is often argued, for instance, that nurses receive low levels of pay because the Health Service relies on their goodwill and concern for patients' welfare to do their job conscientiously. Is this exploitation and, if so, isn't this morally wrong? If so, this turns Titmuss-type arguments for the moral superiority of unpaid (or low paid) donation on its head; for it is saying that the lower the monetary payment the more morally reprehensible is the outcome.

The opposing nature of these arguments can lead us into uncomfortable positions. For in such cases the moral judgements concerned apply to different people. The donor or the low-paid altruistic worker could be viewed as being morally worthy of approval for providing the service concerned for a low reward (or none at all). But the person or institution that pays the low level of reward is being exploitative and could be judged as morally wrong in doing so. In other words, it seems to be morally wrong in such situations to let the altruist behave altruistically. The overall morality of the situation from society's point of view thus becomes very diffiuclt to assess – to say the least.

So where does all this leave us? It is apparent that, in dealing with these issue, we have a potential clash of several moral principles. Paying private providers to perform a public service such as health care may reduce the number of altruistic acts and increase the number of self-interested ones, which would be morally undesirable. However, it may also help to achieve other social ends such as more health care – which, other things being equal, would be morally desirable. And it could be seen as being less exploitative, which would also be desirable on moral grounds.

Now, unless one is prepared to assert unequivocally that one of these principles lexicographically dominates the others – that is, one principle has to be served in all circumstances even if in doing so all other principles are violated – there is no general resolution of this issue. So, if some people believe that the only moral value that has to be served is that concerning the intrinsic moral superiority of altruistic acts (and if they also believe that there are more altruistic public providers than private ones), then they will judge the use of private providers in health care to be morally inferior to the use of public providers – even if the result is less (or worse) health care being provided. If, on the other hand, they believe that society's only concern should be about the level of health care provided and if they also believe that the use of private providers will increase that, then they will support the use of these providers regardless of the impact this has on the stock of altruism in the society. Or, if their only concern to prevent exploitation, then they will support all arrangements that reduce exploitation – even if the result is also less health care and less altruism.

However, in practice, few of us are that black or white in our moral judgements. Most people would recognise that different circumstances yield different answers. For instance, if the result of relying purely on voluntary blood donation, or on low-paid nurses, was that a large number of patients died for a lack of blood available for transfusion or a lack of appropriate nursing care, then we might be prepared to sanction a change in those arrangements, even if the result was less opportunity for the exercise of altruism. If, on the other hand, a switch to less-altruistic modes of provision led to relatively little improvement in outcomes, then we would be less likely to approve of such a change. In the real world, each case has to be examined on its merits and a decision taken as to whether, in that case, the movement towards achieving one principle more than outweighs any movement away from violation of another.

A concluding word

We have seen that the arguments concerning public versus the private provision of health care have moral issues deeply embedded within them and that the moral principles involved may have to be set against one another if the debate is to be resolved. The idea that moral principles or values may have to be 'traded off' is a major insight of modern philosophical discourse.[15] Yet it is alien to many people, especially, it would seem, some of those engaged in the public versus private debate. Ideological stands abound, brooking no compromise and allowing no possibility for trade-off. Yet these kinds of trade-off are inevitable in all policy debate and implementation. In the case of private versus public provision, policy-makers may have to trade-off the moral advantages of public sector altruism against equally valid moral claims relating to outcomes and possible exploitation. In doing so, they would have to examine how much each principle was supported and how much each violated in different cases, and establish their own priorities accordingly. This is not an easy task, and one in which they need to be supported rather than pilloried by moral ideologues on either side.

References

1   Institute for Public Policy Research (IPPR). *Building Better Partnerships: the final report of the Commission on Public Private Partnerships*. London: IPPR, 2001. For an example of a hostile response, see Pollock A, Shaoul J, Rowland D, Player S. *A Response to the IPPR Commission on Public Private Partnerships*. London: The Catalyst Trust, 2001.

2   For further discussion of assumptions concerning public sector motivation and the impact they have had on policy design, see Le Grand J. Knights, knaves or pawns? Human behaviour and social policy. *Journal of Social Policy* 1997; 26: 149–69; and Le Grand J. From knight to knave? Public policy and market incentives. In: Taylor-Gooby P, editor. *Risk, Trust and Welfare*. Houndmills: Macmillan, 2000.

3   It is often claimed that there are other social ends that private provision can also compromise. Equity is particularly vulnerable. In particular, under certain kinds of payment scheme, such as a uniform capitation system, providers have an incentive to 'cream-skim': that is, selecting patients for treatment on the basis of their cheapness to treat rather than their need. Hence, the basic equity principle of equal treatment for equal need is violated. However, this is not intrinsic to private sector provision, for it can be eliminated by suitable risk-adjustment of the payment formulae.

4   Titmuss R. *The Gift Relationship*. London: Allen and Unwin, 1971. Quotations are from new edition; see Oakley A, Ashton J, editors. *Richard Titmuss's The Gift Relationship*. London: LSE Books, 1997.

5   Cooper M, Culyer A. *The Price of Blood*. Hobart Paper 41. London: The Institute of Economic Affairs, 1968.

6   From Oakley A and Ashton J, above.

7   Hobbes T. *Leviathan*. Originally published in 1651. References are to the Penguin Classics edition. London: Penguin Books, 1985.

8   Mandeville B. *The Fable of the Bees*. Originally published in 1714. References are to the Penguin Classics edition. London: Penguin Books, 1989.

9   Butler J. On the relationship between self-love and particular affections. In: Rogers K, editor. *Self-Interest: an anthology of philosophical perspectives*. London: Routledge, 1997: 121–4.

10 Steele J. *Wasted Values: harnessing the commitment of public managers*. London: Public Management Foundation, 1999.

11 Kendall J. Of knights, knaves and merchants: the case of residential care for older people in England in the late 1990s. *Social Policy and Administration* 2001; 35: 360–75.

12 Kendall J, Matosevic T, Forder J, Knapp M, Hardy B, Ware P. *The Motivation of Domiciliary Care Providers in England: new concepts, new findings.* Unpublished paper. London: PSSRU, LSE Health and Social Care, 2001.

13 Taylor-Gooby P, Sylvester S, Calnan M, Manley G. Knights, knaves and gnashers: professional values and private dentistry. *Journal of Social Policy* 2000; 29: 375–95.

14 Berridge V. AIDS and the gift relationship in the UK. In: Oakley A and Ashton J, Chapter 3, above, pp. 20–2.

15 For further discussion, see Barry B. *Political Argument.* London: Routledge and Kegan Paul, 1965; and Le Grand J. *Equity and Choice: an essay in economics and applied philosophy.* London: HarperCollins, 1991.

Chapter 5

A tale of two tribes: the tension between managerial and professional values

David J Hunter

The production of a statement of NHS values has an immediate appeal, especially as it would underpin the Government's commitment to a uniform health system and standardised level of care across the country. But can it serve any useful purpose in a context where there remain significant and deep-seated differences among key groups of stakeholders, especially doctors and managers, in respect of many of the values that such a service might espouse? Moreover, the difficulties in constructing a statement that is of any practical use and goes beyond mere rhetorical superficialities are considerable. Yet they are rarely confronted. The NHS Plan, published in July 2000, is the latest attempt to achieve consensus among the multiple interests in whose hands the fate of the NHS rests.[1] The Plan was formally endorsed by an impressive list of the 'good and the great' from the Health Service community. However, such a show of solidarity did not prevent subsequent criticism of the Plan from various professional groups and anger over some of its proposals.

It is not good enough to talk of NHS values as if there were a common agreed set which was endorsed throughout the Service and by all professional groups. Attempts to achieve consensus about values and to get stakeholder agreement to them overlook the influence of power and politics. The NHS is not, and never has been, a unitary organisation. Rather, it is a coalition of multiple groups, each jostling for supremacy. Furthermore, each group possesses its own particular set of values and these determine whether, and how, it interacts with others. Through such ploys and stratagems, services get, or do not get, delivered. The NHS may be likened to a huge arena in which the various groups play out their power struggles, although these are not always overt. Quite often they take the form of covert interplay between groups with distinctive value systems and cultures. A hierarchy operates among stakeholders, with the medical profession occupying pole position. While it may be possible to overlay these distinctions with a veneer of an agreed set of what might be termed 'meta' or 'high-level' values, for all practical purposes each profession in the NHS behaves according to its own particular core values and beliefs. The agreed meta values have a symbolic function and are largely for public consumption. They do not really serve any useful purpose with regard to providing a corporate framework or bond for NHS staff. Moreover, if they were probed too deeply the internal contradictions and ambiguities would quickly become apparent, as I will discuss below.

The malaise and dis-ease evident throughout the NHS is widespread, and seemingly getting worse, as measured by rising rates of staff absenteeism, early retirement, and poor recruitment and retention of staff. The possible connection between these indicators of a sick organisation may, at least in part, be a product of the absence of a common set of values both within the NHS and between it and its users. It is not enough that new investment is going into the NHS following years of underinvestment. There is the vexed question of how that investment is to be used and to what purpose. The issues here are more contentious and conflictual. Is the NHS intent on reducing waiting lists and using hospital beds more intensively? Or does it seek to develop primary care in innovative ways that could, through managing demand more effectively, avoid much unnecessary hospital treatment? Does it want more doctors and nurses in order to deal with a growing workload but to continue with a 'more of the same' approach? Or does it want the next generation of doctors and nurses to behave and work in quite different ways? For example, will NHS staff train together and work as partners rather than as separate professional sparring partners, each trained in his or her own silo with its particular values and culture? As a society, do we really want national uniformity in terms of what the NHS does? Or do we want a service that is customised to local needs and circumstances, which probably means being more tolerant of diversity? It may be that we do not have a clear or fixed view about the appropriate balance between a NHS based on a 'one size fits all' mentality and one that is more sensitive to local variations and community needs.

Questions like these have no simple or easy answers. Nor perhaps should they. They may be examples of the 'unwinnable dilemmas of social policy'.[2] It is the essence of public policy and public services that such 'wicked issues' are what distinguish them from private sector businesses and comparatively simple transactions in the marketplace.[3] The NHS contains within itself numerous contradictions and multiple objectives. Not all of these are mutually reinforcing or reconcilable. Balancing, and negotiating among, the different interests and values are, after all, what is unique about public management. With the Government prepared to privatise much of the delivery of health care, along the lines of its policies in education and transport, it raises further complexity and complications in respect of how private sector values compare and contrast with public sector ones.

The remainder of this chapter considers the current condition of the NHS in terms of the all-pervading sense of unease that is evident, and examines its possible causes centring on the notion of tribalism – a key feature of the NHS. Among the tribes there is little sense of common purpose or unity behind a set of shared values. At best, there is a veneer of consensus over what the NHS stands for. These issues are considered in the context of the tension between managerialism and professionalism. A final section explores whether there is any prospect of an accommodation between these two distinct ways of looking at the NHS, or whether it is right that there remains a healthy creative tension between the two distinct value positions.

'Doing better, feeling worse'

A US political scientist, Aaron Wildavsky, coined the pithy phrase 'doing better, feeling worse' to describe the paradox whereby putting more resources into health care had the effect of ratcheting up yet further expectations among both staff and public that could not be met.[4] These simply triggered calls for yet more investment. The same paradoxical effect is evident in the NHS. Despite the significant new investment in the NHS, the 'feel-good' factor is strikingly absent. It was probably always thus. Following a spell as health minister in the early 1960s, Enoch Powell produced a perceptive and eloquent account of the structural weakness of the NHS.[5] As he described it, the NHS was the helpless victim of the annual clamour for resources and those who shouted loudest, or denigrated the Service the most, tended to do well out of the allocation process. The incentive, perversely, was to run down and criticise the NHS rather than to point to its achievements.

But the problem goes deeper and touches on the values question. The IPPR/King's Fund report on NHS values poses the issues clearly.[6] It asserts that NHS values are increasingly muddled and are neither mutually supporting or reinforcing. Internal contradictions and conflicts abound. Whether it is possible in that setting actually to manage a set of trade-offs sensibly is unclear – the values may be so distinctive that it may not be easy to have an optimising approach. Should this be so surprising, given the contested nature of much of what the NHS does and how it does it? The more puzzling question may be why we are so exercised about the absence of a common set of values. And why should so many commentators and others subscribe to the view that there ought to be a common set of values? If such a set were genuinely to inform how decisions were made, then that might constitute a sufficiently persuasive argument in its favour. But for the reasons already given, that seems an unlikely outcome. What, then, is the value of an agreed statement of values which would probably have to exist at a level of abstraction that would be likely to deny their utility for all practical purposes?

Proponents of a statement of values would probably argue that the issues with which a values statement would attempt to deal have only recently surfaced in the public domain and are now given painstaking and forensic attention by the media and members of the public. As long as the NHS was a somewhat opaque, if not wholly impenetrable, organisation there was probably not an issue to be confronted because decisions were not particularly transparent or explicit and the matter of values did not receive much attention as a consequence.

However, a side effect of being explicit and transparent under the twin spotlights of a more critical media and a restive, if yet to be empowered, public is that it exposes the internal contradictions within the NHS and puts them in a stark light. Whatever their implications for the health of democracy, these contradictions may prove irreconcilable in the spotlight of publicity and public attention.

As noted above, the NHS is riven with divisions and disagreements, and there is considerable paradox and potential, though often latent, conflict between health and health care; primary care and general practice; individualism and collectivism; patient and citizen; and top-down and bottom-up models of policy-making and implementation.

It is little wonder therefore that the high-level values New identifies for the NHS (see Box 5.1) are in conflict with each other when there is an absence of consensus on the way forward for the NHS (see Box 5.2).

BOX 5.1 NHS VALUES

- Health
- Universalism
- Equity
- Democracy
- Choice
- Respect for human dignity
- Public service
- Efficiency

BOX 5.2 VALUE CONFLICTS

- Choice v. equity
- Equity v. efficiency
- Democracy v. equity
- Efficiency v. democracy
- Efficiency v. universalism
- Health v. non-NHS values

The absence of clarity of purpose in the NHS, coupled with various internal contradictions and conflicts, constitute key sources of the malaise and poor morale evident in the Service. These, in turn, may reflect a deeper problem, namely, a lack of confidence about the NHS from within, which inevitably fuels negative public perceptions of it externally. Whether or not there exists an actual NHS 'crisis' is open to argument. More likely, the 'crisis' has been manufactured by a steady stream of adverse media invective and by a Government which appears not to believe in or trust those providing or managing health services, and whom it perceives as cautionary fatalists rather than as thrusting modernisers. A consequence is a serious loss of confidence evident both inside and outside the Service.

For all its alleged support for the NHS, the Government seems to regard much of it as 'Old Labour' and not 'New Labour'. Notwithstanding the NHS Plan's espousal of a public service ethos, it has not prevented the Government from applauding the virtues of private sector management skills in its proposal for privately run 'health factories' to perform routine operations. Is there not a contradiction here which has it origins in a fundamental clash of values? Are the two stances reconcilable? Will the championing of the private sector not further erode the notion of a public service ethic at precisely the moment when the Government wishes to restore and strengthen it?

It might be that value trade-offs could be achieved if there were a greater degree of unity and common purpose throughout the NHS among those who manage and provide health care. Yet, for all the Government's attempts to brand the NHS as a 'national' enterprise and ensure that it delivers a high-quality standardised product across the country to overcome charges of a postcode lottery in care, the reality remains a highly diverse and pluralistic health care system. No progress can be made on the values question without an appreciation of this complex system.

Tribalism in the NHS jungle

No one in the NHS seems happy these days. The dilemma is probably not confined to the NHS, although the problems seem particularly acute there. Low morale among staff is nothing new. What is different is the scale of the problem and the fact that it now affects the total workforce. In the past, while some groups may have harboured grievances, others fared rather better. This no longer appears to be the case, with every professional group simultaneously feeling a deep sense of malaise and demotivation. An editorial in the *British Medical Journal* posed the question: why are doctors unhappy?[7] It suggested the causes were multiple, although one in particular was highlighted – 'the mismatch between what doctors were trained for and what they are required to do'. Trained in some specialty or field of medicine, 'doctors find themselves spending more time thinking about issues like management, improvement, finance, law, ethics, and communication'.

Managers are no less unhappy with their lot, although perhaps they attract less sympathy from a public that is ever sceptical (or ignorant) of their added value. Whereas in the Thatcher era of the NHS internal market, managers generally felt empowered and in charge of events, they now appear cowed and beleaguered functionaries in a system that is more politicised than ever and whose political heads regard themselves as its leaders. Far from being engaged in shaping policy and its implementation, managers feel excluded and marginalised.

In a situation where there is universal unease among the key stakeholders about the state of the NHS, it seems curious that there has not been organised dissent of some description. But with the exception of some modest flexing of muscles among revolting GPs, nothing has occurred on a grand scale and there has been no backlash that cuts across the professions. Were the NHS a truly integrated, corporate entity whose employees subscribed to an agreed set of values, perhaps things would be different. But such a sense of collective cohesion does not exist in the NHS. As noted above, it is a loose coalition of interest groups, each in possession of its own carefully preserved view of the world. The reasons for such pluralism go deep and have their roots in the origins of the NHS.

The NHS is like no other organisation in the public or private sectors. Although there are some parallels with other organisations which have a strong professional component, like education and social work, and its equivalent in the creative arts (e.g. the BBC and other media), the status and privileges traditionally enjoyed by the medical profession are unparalleled. The NHS's essential distinctiveness lies in the fact that it is a split organisation with a bureaucratic component and a professional component.[8] This split organisational form underlies many of the management problems and tensions in the NHS which have persisted almost from the outset. These, in turn, have their origins in the value clashes between the two components. The organisational form assumed by the NHS, and the distribution of power and authority within it, are deeply affected by the doctors' special (some would say collusive) relationship with their patients. Other professional groups, notably nurses, have their special features, too, but the medical profession has had, and for the most part continues to have, a unique authority. As Rowbottom[9] puts it:

> the position of doctors ... presents a fascinating, and possibly unique, situation to any student of organisation. Never have so many highly influential figures been found in such an equivocal position – neither wholly of, nor wholly divorced from, the organisation which they effectively dominate (p.73).

The relationship between the medical profession and managers is characterised by two different sets of aims and objectives, as well as different values. In essence, doctors insist upon treating individual patients in the manner they see to be in the patients' best interests and regard themselves as being accountable to the patients they serve and to their own conscience.

In contrast, managers are concerned with the operation of the NHS as a whole and with ensuring that resources benefit the needs of a particular population or community rather than simply those of any single individual. This tension lies at the heart of the management challenge within the NHS and accounts for the ambivalence many doctors feel towards the management function. It is an ambivalence which has been compounded by the particular models and styles of management which have been introduced at various stages over the past 25 years or so.

Other factors and influences are at work. Lee-Potter[10] may have put his finger on it when he states with commendable candour:

> *Doctors are unavoidably elitist. They have been used to being amongst the brightest in their schools, they have had to work longer and harder while at university ... The lot of a junior doctor is a hard one, and it does not get much easier during the rest of a medical career, whether in hospital or general practice. From this point of view, the path to chief executive of a trust hospital, on a salary equal to or higher than that of a consultant with at least a 'B' merit award ... looks much easier. If the truth were told it probably is* (p.249).

There is some empirical evidence to provide substance to these contrasting views, found among doctors and managers respectively. In fact, the picture is more complicated because nurses have their own value position. Degeling and colleagues undertook a comparative study of professional sub-cultures in English and Australian hospitals.[11] The subcultures comprised five occupational groups: medical clinicians, medical managers, nurse clinicians, nurse managers and lay managers. The study elicited views on the following themes

- key health care issues
- strategies for dealing with hospital resource issues
- interconnections between the clinical and resource dimensions of care
- the causes of clinical practice variation
- who should be involved in setting clinical standards
- the forms of knowledge on which clinical standards should be based
- how clinical units should be managed
- the accountability and autonomy of medical and nursing clinicians.

The views obtained were placed alongside the four elements comprising the reform agenda in each country that followed a similar trajectory.[12] These require health care professionals and managers to:

- recognise interconnections between the clinical and financial dimensions of care

- participate in processes which will increase the systemisation and integration of clinical work and bring it within the ambit of work process control
- accept the multidisciplinary and team-based nature of clinical service provision and accept the need to establish structures and practices capable of supporting this
- adopt a perspective which balances clinical autonomy with transparent accountability.

The findings point to significant profession-based differences on each of the four elements of the reform agenda. For example, on efforts to gain recognition of interconnections between the clinical and resource dimensions of care, the data suggest a continuum of views ranging from a 'clinical purist' stance to a 'financial realist' stance. Clinical purists proceed from the view that efforts to link clinical and resource issues, and make transparent the resource implications of clinical practice, will be detrimental to care. For them, patient need as determined by clinical judgement should be the only determinant of how resources are allocated and that clinicians should not be held directly responsible for the resource implications of their practices. In contrast, financial realists argue that clinical decisions are also resource decisions and that the two are inherently interconnected.

Similarly, with respect to work process control, the data show a continuum of views between respondents who favour increasing the systemisation and integration of clinical work and those who are opposed. Included here are the development and implementation of clinical pathways, utilisation review, quality assurance processes and clinical audits. Respondents whose work concentrates on direct patient care (i.e. medical clinicians and nurse clinicians) are inclined to a clinical purist stance. On the other hand, whereas lay managers are strongly financial realists, nurse managers are only marginally so. For their part, and in keeping with their location at the boundary of clinical and managerial identities, the responses of medical managers reflect the importance of their pre-existing clinical affiliations over their newly assigned managerial responsibilities. Medical managers marginally favour autonomous clinical judgement over work process control. Whereas they recognise that all clinical decisions are resource decisions, their rejection of work process control methods means medical managers deny themselves the structures and methods they need to manage these interconnections.

Finally, the same dissonance is evident in efforts to promote more team-based approaches to clinical work. They require the resolution of medical clinicians' individualistic (i.e. anti-team) stance, as compared with nurse clinicians' collective conception of clinical work. The data show that medical managers are likely to join with medical clinicians in objecting to moves on this front.

These findings clearly demonstrate the barriers that face those seeking to introduce changes in the delivery of health care. For those changes to happen there needs to be a common sense of purpose and a set of core values shared by the key stakeholders. These prior conditions do not exist. All attempts to impose managerial controls on clinical work are doomed to failure unless a different approach to managing change is adopted. This has been the unequivocal lesson from recent moves to tighten the managerial grip on the NHS.[13]

A constant theme running through successive reorganisations of the NHS since the mid-1970s has been the search for improved management. The search has been accompanied by growing centralisation, despite occasional lapses into decentralisation. As Hoggett observes more generally in the restructuring of the public sector in Britain, elements of decentralised, hands-off, market-based approaches to delivering public services have been 'dwarfed by visible elements of centralisation ... and the extended use of hands-on systems of performance management creating a form of "evaluative state"'.[14]

The excessive degree of centralisation and formalisation, which shows no sign of abating, has had unforeseen consequences on the dynamics of the NHS. As Jenkins puts it: 'the centralisation of the NHS left an uneasy feeling that a professional relationship of trust between patient and doctor and hospital and community had been broken' (p.88).[15] He contrasts the monster (he is referring to the NHS internal market) created by Thatcher and health secretary Kenneth Clarke with Aneurin Bevan's original model for the NHS: 'His health service was concerned simply with offering doctors and nurses an administrative apparatus "for them freely to use in accordance with their training for the benefit of the people of the country"' (ibid, p.86).

Bevan's model was the profession-dominated NHS which survived largely intact until the first half of the 1980s, when the model was questioned by a businessman, Roy Griffiths, brought in by the government of the day to advise on the future management of the NHS. Griffiths sought to strengthen management and to shift the emphasis, and eventually the balance of power, from producers to consumers, in line with commercial practice. He was tapping into a trend that was becoming established internationally. The tenets of what became known as 'new public management' (NPM) entered the public sector reform lexicon in many countries almost simultaneously.[16] Of particular importance was the emphasis in NPM on standard setting, performance management, and target setting in the sphere of professional influence. Also important was the stress on private sector management and the move away from the traditional public service ethic.

Over several decades, the upshot of the various management reforms in the NHS on the medical profession has been closer bureaucratic control of its activities. Hence the observation reported earlier that a cause of unhappiness among doctors is the intrusion of management into their working lives in ways neither foreseen nor regarded as helpful or in line with professional beliefs and values. Nevertheless, the perception of a profession whose autonomy is under threat from politicians and managers, as well as from health services researchers intent upon challenging medical practice variations, is real and can only add to the unhappiness that doctors feel.

Moreover, the market-style experiment introduced in the first half of the 1990s had a corrosive effect on the hitherto 'high-trust' relationships between doctors and managers and between doctors and patients.[17] It was not simply the talk of markets and competition in health care that many professionals found offensive and inappropriate (indeed, many managers shared these perceptions but their opposition remained muted since the majority of their colleagues welcomed the growing influence and power accorded them), but the entire panoply of management systems and controls, which appeared to be founded on notions of distrust and focused almost exclusively on cost improvements and efficiency gains. Whatever its shortcomings, and there were many, the pre-1984 NHS was based on 'high-trust' relationships in which the parties involved observed mutual obligations which were not precisely defined. That these relationships may not always have been evident in practice does not negate the assumptions underpinning the management style then operating.

In contrast, the post-1984 and 1991 changes replaced a consensus model with one based on the management of conflict.[18] The new model implied low trust relationships: every transaction and encounter must be defined, codified, documented, formalised and transformed into a quasi-contractual relationship. In his seminal study of labour management issues, Fox[19] defines 'high-trust' relationships as ones in which the participants share (or have similar) ends and values; have a diffuse sense of long-term obligation; offer support without calculating the cost or expecting an immediate return; communicate freely and openly with one another; are prepared to trust the other and risk their own fortunes in the other party; give the benefit of the doubt in relation to motives and goodwill if there are problems. In contrast, 'low-trust' relationships are ones in which the participants have divergent goals; have explicit expectations which must be reciprocated through balanced exchanges; carefully calculate the costs and benefits of any concession made; restrict and screen communications in their own separate interests; attempt to minimise their dependence on the other's discretion; are suspicious about mistakes or failures, attributing them to ill will or default and invoke sanctions.

The arrival of markets in the NHS, together with a particular brand of hard-line managerialism,[20] seriously eroded 'high-trust' relationships. A link can be traced to the increasing subjugation of doctors to the edicts of the new managerialism, with their stress on control and accountability, and doctors' growing frustration at seeing their power base or sphere of influence challenged. Under New Labour, relationships have not improved and may in fact have deteriorated. Despite the Government's insistence that the market is dead and that 'joined-up' policy and partnership working are back in favour, few feel assured by the Government's aggressive top-down management style.

The concerns of the medical profession can, with some justification, be understood as no more than a display of naked protectionism, but they are nevertheless understandable and not entirely without foundation. They cannot summarily be dismissed as being of no consequence or substance. As Pollitt argues, the new orthodoxy of managerialism amounted to 'a set of beliefs and practices, at the core of which burns the seldom-tested assumption that better management will prove an effective solvent for a wide range of economic and social ills'.[21]

Compounding the hostility to management in the NHS and contributing to the erosion of trust between doctors and managers is doctors' perception of managers as the agents of government ministers rather than as a group of enablers and facilitators that exists primarily to support doctors. Though managers may have their own values, along the lines described earlier, they are increasingly perceived as the handmaidens of ministers and progressively incapable of acting independently according to their values, unless these happen to accord with those of their political masters. Ironically, given their opposition to the NHS concept in the first place, in recent years doctors have come to see themselves as the sole remaining guardians of the founding principles of the NHS, with managers cast as the NHS's greatest enemy.[22] When the NHS started life, managers were not expected to have a voice or be assertive. Their task was to create an environment for doctors to practice medicine. Now doctors see managers ruling the roost, with clinical work subordinated to the ever-growing demands of clinical governance and financial management.

As the power balance between doctors and managers has shifted inexorably towards managers, doctors have in general become increasingly vociferous and strident in their condemnation of the NHS in general and the cult of managerialism in particular. Joining the ranks of hospital doctors who have been subjected to this state of affairs for many years are GPs who, until recently, remained untouched. But with the development of new primary care organisations, GPs are now being subjected to exactly the same style of managerialism. As independent contractors with a particular conception of their relationship with the NHS, few are taking kindly to what they consider to be unacceptable intrusion into their professional lives. As Gray and Jenkins conclude, the nature of power and politics in the NHS has been altered 'at the expense of the professionals and to the advantage of the managers' (p.29).[23]

Despite the encroachment by management into medicine, its impact on practice and behaviour should not be overstated. The micro-management of medical work is weak and will probably remain so until doctors manage themselves and their work.[24] Simpson and Smith, who argue that 'all clinicians must know something about management, even if it is to be able followers rather than leaders' (p.1637), endorse the point.[25] But not all doctors feel so inclined. Lee-Potter, a former chairman of the BMA Council, maintains that 'relatively few' doctors actually want to be managers.[26]

His assessment receives strong support from a survey of young doctors' views of their core values conducted by the BMA.[27] The survey found considerable hostility towards management, whose apparently conflicting culture and different ethos and value base, doctors believed, prevented them from practising medicine to the benefit of their patients. The respondents were particularly concerned about the demands to maintain throughput and numbers, and to account for their time. The young doctors surveyed saw management as becoming increasingly intrusive and aggressive in questioning the commitment of doctors through their working practices. Many felt 'hassle' from management to speed up their consultations and to see more patients. The view was expressed that consultants were becoming less and less empowered because they are becoming more like 'technical monkeys'. A great cultural divide existed between doctors and managers, particularly when it came to understanding the core values of the medical profession. Doctors presented a bleak picture of misunderstanding and territorial separation, which illustrated the width of the gulf between them and managers. Managers were perceived as individuals who 'don't know what we do and they don't want to know either' (ibid, p.8).

Those interviewed did not feel they would increase their autonomy by taking on a more managerial role. Managers were seen as a different species. As one respondent put it: 'managers don't share the same ethics as us, and so it's assumed that if you cross the road and become a manager, you've lost some of those values that are held dear to doctors' (ibid, p.11). And therein lies the nub of the problem. Such perceptions inevitably framed and coloured discussions of whether doctors should or could take on more managerial roles. Some respondents referred to colleagues who had taken on more managerial responsibilities as 'traitors' or as having 'copped out'. But there was a preference for dealing with managers who had been clinicians because their judgement could be trusted. Significantly, this trust was mostly based on the perception that the manager with a medical background still shared the same core values as the doctors, while managers with no such background were perceived to have a different value system. Despite this perception, some of those interviewed gave examples of the ways in which the core values of medical managers could be overruled by management, particularly on issues of quality compared with numbers.

Finding a way forward

Not all management incursions into clinical work can be condemned outright or rejected as having no relevance or useful public purpose. As Allen notes in her report on the BMA survey of young doctors, many of the demands for greater accountability, measurable outputs and more throughput are well founded and have sought to remove some restrictive practices. Not all professionals perform in ways that uphold the high ideals and standards set for them. The privileges they enjoy can be abused in ways, and appear self-serving and protectionist. Other aspects of the management revolution, however, 'have succeeded only in demotivating and demoralising professionals who have sought to maintain core values in a world which has become increasingly wedded to efficiency and the management culture' (ibid, p.14).

The BMA survey emphasised the unanimity over the cultural divide between doctors and managers, which was proving wholly counterproductive and stress inducing. The two groups occupied quite separate and distinct worlds. While younger doctors acknowledged the need to modernise the profession, they remained wedded to a commitment to provide competence, care and compassion for those in need. But they were resistant to what many saw as a managerial takeover which, if it succeeded, would almost certainly threaten their values and practice.

It is easy to fall into the trap of shooting the messenger. There are many managers who are equally unhappy about their political masters' and mistresses' expectations of them as public servants. They feel resentful at the constant stress placed upon numbers, whether it is the length of waiting lists, the number of patients treated, the number of beds available, or the balancing of the books. Of course, such bottom-line issues are important, but these seem to be the only things that matter. Even when there is expressed commitment to quality issues and to strategic initiatives which seek to achieve a better balance between providing health care and improving the overall health of local communities, all evident during the early years of the Government's term of office, in reality they count for little and are not sacking offences for chief executives. These managers are frustrated by the obsession of politicians with input targets and efficiency measures that have little to say about effectiveness and outcomes.

Given the unhappiness apparent in equal measure among front-line professionals and managers, perhaps therein lies hope of a resolution in the stand-off between the two camps. There is a need for an honest dialogue between the two groups. This might entail a new beginning, since the root of the problem may lie in the type and style of management that has evolved within the NHS. It may be inappropriate for the task, as clinicians and managers are beginning to appreciate. The cult of managerialism prevalent in the NHS reflects accounting rather than clinical or quality-of-service criteria. Accommodating these two sets of values is unlikely to prove straightforward. But, as Lee-Potter and others have argued, some form of accommodation must be found between managers and doctors. One way forward may be to integrate the training of managers with that of doctors, at some stage in their careers, in order to bring them closer together: 'The intention would not be to turn doctors into managers or vice versa, but simply to familiarise each group with the other's priorities, skills and problems faced, and help to achieve better teamwork and thus a better health service' (p.250).[28]

Hope of finding some accommodation between clinicians and managers also lies in resisting the temptation to polarise the two sides. The reality is more complex and, conceivably, hopeful in terms of future developments aimed at finding some accommodation between front-line professionals and managers. Many doctors accept the need to manage resources optimally and support the drive to base decisions on knowledge and evidence of effectiveness.

Some hope for the future may also lie in the work of Degeling and his colleagues on professional sub-cultures reported earlier. They argue that a prerequisite for sustainable change in the way professions and managers operate and work to find common ground is to identify champions for change. From their research, they conclude that the appointment of clinical directors suggests that medical and nurse managers are best placed to support change. However, their willingness and ability to become involved in implementing reform will depend on the extent to which they have developed a clear understanding of their newly acquired identities in ways that distinguish them from their clinical colleagues. Without this, their capacity to mediate between clinical and managerial conceptions of clinical work will be limited. Degeling and his colleagues are not wholly optimistic about the ability of medical managers to assume the position required of them if the reform agenda is to be achieved. Their research shows that 15 years after the commencement of health care reform, 32 per cent of medical managers in the sample continued to share common ground with their clinical colleagues. The development of a distinct medical managerial perspective remains, at best, fragile.

But the prospects are not entirely devoid of hope. The data also show that above all other staff groups, nurse managers are the most supportive of the reform agenda. Furthermore, the data show that 16 per cent of medical clinicians, together with 12 per cent of medical managers, indicated that they believe team-based clinical unit management and involvement in resource-based clinical unit management will enhance their autonomy; support strategies will improve work systemisation and service integration; and support a team-based work process control model for clinical unit management. These respondents have distanced themselves from their medical colleagues and it is therefore within their ranks that the champions of reform are likely to be found.

However, there are two important provisos which will determine the final outcome. First, the capacity of managers to effect change in clinical practice is severely limited as a consequence of the centrality of the medical profession as a defining feature of health care organisations. In short, efforts to extend and strengthen the role of management in health care settings signal substantial shifts in the values that underpin management/clinician relations. As has been reported here, the successful enactment of these changes in successive reorganisations over the years has proved problematic.[29]

Second, there is accumulating evidence, also reported here, of the way that management's standing among medical and nursing clinicians is adversely affected by pressure from central government to meet financial and activity performance targets. Such a mechanistic, reductionist view of the management task is at odds with what many managers would regard as an equally, if not more, important job of managing for improved quality and health outcomes. The politicisation of management and the consequent distortion of the values managers might otherwise wish to uphold is a serious obstacle to achieving a set of shared values.[30]

It will not be easy to introduce an approach to managing health care that is based on a common value base among professionals and managers. It is likely to be dismissed as yet another management fad. Health care staff, already cynical and demoralised, may view the new approach with considerable scepticism and it could exacerbate the climate of distrust which characterises relations between medical, nursing and managerial staff. However, though very real, these constraints must not be allowed to vitiate the attempt to align the values of the various groups involved in the health care enterprise. Only in this way can their contribution to improving the health of populations be optimally harnessed.

References

1   Secretary of State for Health. *The NHS Plan: a plan for investment; a plan for reform*. Cm 4818-I. London: Stationery Office, 2000.
2   Heclo H. Social politics and policy impacts. In: Holden Jr. M, Dresang D L, editors. *What Government Does*. Beverly Hills: Sage, 1975.
3   Stewart J. Advance or retreat: from the traditions of public administration to the new public management and beyond. *Public Policy and Administration* 1998; 13 (4): 12–27.
4   Wildavsky A. *The Art and Craft of Policy Analysis*. London: Macmillan, 1979.
5   Powell J E. *Medicine and Politics*. London: Pitman Medical, 1966.
6   New B. *A Good-Enough Service: values, trade-offs and the NHS*. London: Institute for Public Policy Research and King's Fund, 1999.
7   Smith R. Why are doctors so unhappy? *BMJ* 2001; 322: 1073–4.

8   Susser M, Watson W. *Sociology in Medicine*. London: Oxford University Press, 1971.

9   Rowbottom R *et al*. *Hospital Organisation*. London: Heinemann, 1973.

10 Lee-Potter J. *A Damn Bad Business: the NHS deformed*. London: Gollancz, 1997.

11 Degeling P, Kennedy J, Hill M. Do professional subcultures set limits to hospital reform? *Clinician in Management* 1998; 7: 89–98.

12 Degeling P, Hunter D J, Dowdeswell B. Changing health care systems. *Journal of Integrated Care Pathways* 2001 (in press).

13 Hunter D J. Managing the NHS. In: Appleby J, Harrison A, editors. *Health Care UK, Winter 2000*. London: King's Fund, 2000.

14 Hoggett P. New modes of control in the public service. *Public Administration* 1996; 69 (1): 9–32.

15 Jenkins S. *Accountable to None: the Tory nationalisation of Britain*. London: Hamish Hamilton, 1995.

16 Hood C. A public management for all seasons? *Public Administration* 1991; 69 (1): 3–19.

17 Harrison S, Lachmann P. *Towards a High-Trust NHS*. London: Institute for Public Policy Research, 1996.

18 Day P, Klein R. The mobilisation of consent versus the management of conflict: decoding the Griffiths Report. *BMJ* 1983; 287: 1213–16.

19 Fox A. *Beyond Contract: work, power, and trust relations*. London: Faber and Faber, 1974.

20 Burns T. Introduction to Second Edition. In: Burns T, Stalker G, editors. *Management of Innovation*. Oxford: Oxford University Press, 1994.

21 Pollitt C. *Managerialism and the Public Sector: cuts or cultural change?* 2nd edition. Oxford: Blackwell, 1993.

22 Wall A. The NHS: who is attacking, who is defending? *Health Care Analysis* 1996; 4: 328–31.

23 Gray A, Jenkins B. Public management and the NHS. In: Glynn J, Perkins D, editors. *Managing Health Care*. London: Saunders, 1995.

24 Burns T, 1996, above.

25 Simpson J, Smith R. Why healthcare systems need medical managers. *BMJ* 1997; 314: 1636–7.

26 Lee-Potter J, 1997, above.

27 Allen I. *Committed but Critical: an examination of young doctors' views of their core values*. London: British Medical Association, 1997.

28 Lee-Potter J, 1997, above.

29 Hunter D J. *Coping with Uncertainty: policy and politics in the National Health Service*. Chichester: Wiley & Sons, 1980; and Hunter D J. Medicine. In: Laffin M, editor. *Beyond Bureaucracy? The Professions in the Contemporary Public Sector*. Aldershot: Ashgate, 1998.

30 Calman K, Hunter D J, May A. *Things Can Only Get Better: a commentary on implementing the NHS Plan*. Durham: University of Durham Business School, 2001.

Chapter 6

Democracy is king … or mother knows best?

Pamela Charlwood

How should decisions be made about health issues and who can claim legitimacy as a decision-maker? A highly persuasive case can be made, particularly on issues affecting people's health, that consumers should have a powerful say. This principle would be argued by civil rights campaigners, and is frequently backed up by politicians and has been strengthened by the implementation of the Human Rights Act. But if public opinion is at odds with views which are based on evidence from research and scientific knowledge – or which may arise from pragmatic considerations such as the requirements of training, whether staff can be recruited or simple affordability – how much weight should it carry? What is more, the government of the day may have policies which are in line with scientific evidence but not popular opinion, or vice versa. Finally, in listening to public opinion, those who make decisions on health issues must also consider people whose voices are less easily heard than the more audible constituencies, whose cases prove most attractive to the media. Those who are less frequently heard may include people with learning difficulties, people suffering mental distress, older people and children, and it is important for decision-makers to demonstrate that their interests and arguments have been weighed as seriously as those whose causes are more audible and persuasive. In this chapter I will first reflect in more detail on these trade-offs; second, I will briefly consider a number of more radical approaches to democratic practice; finally, I propose some principles for guiding decision-makers when faced with conflicting demands in a modern democratic nation.

Democracy versus other values

In very many cases, public opinion may support a wholly sensible and appropriate course of action, and it would be deeply patronising to suggest otherwise. However, there are a variety of circumstances in which public opinion and experience may be at odds with the views of appointed decision-makers or 'experts'.

First, there are instances where it may feel as though the public and the professionals are simply from different tribes, speaking different languages which are mutually incomprehensible. Many health authorities, for example, will have encountered the public outcry at the loss or potential loss of a much-loved single-handed GP who has practised within a community for many years. The health authority and, indeed, clinical colleagues may be able to offer evidence of lack of services, lack of up-to-date knowledge or training, lack of audit of outcomes and lack of peer support. But, even after the extreme case of Dr Harold Shipman, patients may well continue to champion such an individual, finding such criticism at odds with the personal relationship which may have been built up over years if not generations.

Further examples can be offered of hospital services which, on any objective measure of service quality and outcomes, might be shown to be less good for patients than they should expect: paediatric surgery, carried out by non-specialists many miles from the specialist centre; complex cancer surgery, carried out by generalists; an accident & emergency department losing training accreditation and staffed mainly by locums. These examples represent a particular challenge to health decision-makers. Should they tell the public that the service they have been receiving is unsafe or at least of an unacceptable quality? This may well conflict with public perceptions of the service and also raises challenging questions in relation to the politics and public relations around the issue. 'Health chiefs admit service is unsafe' is not a headline which many of us would particularly welcome.

A second category where public and professional views might differ is where the issue is complex and genuinely difficult to understand. The location of services for cleft lip and palate might be one such example, where the national expert group has striven for more than two years to suggest a configuration of services which will meet the rigorous standards which have been set, but will also meet the needs of people in the predominantly urban regions of London and the West Midlands, as well as the rural region of the South West. In this example, the people of Devon and Dorset, who have hitherto received a surgical service for cleft lip and palate in their local areas, will now perceive that they are being offered the prospect of travelling to a service in Salisbury, Oxford, Bristol or even Birmingham. Since the finer points of the arguments around critical mass and clinical relationships have been somewhat opaque to health professionals, it is only reasonable to acknowledge that the general public might find them totally incomprehensible.

A third area for potential difficulty is where different democratic representatives seem to come into conflict, specifically where the policies and priorities of central government differ from the position taken by local authorities. The members of a local authority, for instance, may find the current Government's proposals to establish Care Trusts, with responsibility for both health and social services, unacceptable because of the lack of (local) democratic accountability of these proposed bodies. Central government, however, has brought in legislation to establish Care Trusts in a way which would not only draw together these interdependent services but would also, arguably, bring social services under far more direct control of the centre. However, it is difficult to argue simply that such actions are undemocratic – central government has its own strong national mandate, in this case the result of two resounding general election victories gained on a platform of reforming public services. The centre–local debate over democratic accountability has yet further manifestations: there are those who argue passionately for the introduction of direct election of members of health statutory bodies; others would shudder at the prospect of health becoming even more of a political football than it is now.

In a fourth example, local democracy may also throw up apparently inequitable or unfair outcomes. In a health authority area which encompasses four unitary authorities, for instance, one local authority, Bristol City Council, recently put its money where its mouth was in terms of the democratic process, and in early 2001 held a referendum asking the voters what they wanted to happen to their Council Tax. To peg the Council Tax would mean a reduction in services; a modest increase would hold services at their current level; a larger increase would enable improvements to be made. Forty per cent of those eligible to vote did so, with 53 per cent of them voting for the 'no increase – reduce services' option. The voters had stated their preference and so education and social services, amongst other departments, are implementing major reductions in services for children and older people. Across the road, in the neighbouring local authority area, councillors were less democratic and services are being sustained.

This example opens up the question of when local democracy becomes a 'vox pop' which has limited sympathy for – and possibly limited understanding of – the needs of the most vulnerable people in society. In rather similar circumstances, an equivalent popular poll might show that the majority of people found it easier to be sympathetic to some groups of people rather than others – for example, cancer patients, premature babies and people waiting for heart surgery, rather than drug misusers, alcoholics and people with sexually transmitted diseases. Should the official decision-makers, therefore, enter the debate as the champions of those whose case is deemed less attractive?

Radical options

A number of radical approaches to decision-making have been put forward – in particular referendums and citizens' juries – and each needs to be tested against these considerations. So too does an approach which could be described as more centralised decision-making, exemplified by the role of the National Institute for Clinical Excellence (NICE) and introduced in the interests of achieving greater consistency.

On the question of referendums, three concerns arise. First, have the issues – and their implications – been well enough described, understood and debated, so that the vote cast is genuinely well informed? Second, is there a reasonable representation of those likely to be most affected in the voters, or is there a disproportionate showing from the more articulate middle classes? Third, the voter who puts the cross in the box does not then have to take any responsibility for the consequences of his or her action. He or she can remain anonymous and free to applaud, criticise or remain silent as the result of the vote becomes a reality.

Citizens' juries are exempt from some of these potential criticisms, since their deliberations and decisions are likely to be in the public domain. Thus far, the issues put to citizens' juries by health bodies have been quite clearly focused, tending to relate to single issues or decisions, attractively untroubled by the infinite messiness and complexity of real life. Could it ever be reasonable to delegate to such a panel the whole range of dilemmas with which a health authority or PCT Board must grapple, further intensified by the targets and guidance issued by central government? The temporary jurors, too – like their counterparts in the judicial system – are not required to implement and live with the consequences of their decisions, but can retire to lay anonymity once their job is done. And who would be subject to judicial review if a challenge were brought on the results of the deliberations of a citizens' jury? Surely it would be the statutory health body rather than the temporary jury.

Within the NHS, there have been undeniable variations in policy and priorities between different geographical areas, giving rise to real concerns –

and much media coverage – of what has been described as 'postcode prescribing' or 'rationing'. Part of this has arisen from different interpretations of the scientific evidence on both clinical and cost-effectiveness, as well as different judgements about local priorities. It might have been expected that the advent of the NICE would help to overcome the dilemmas and debates about what the evidence really says and what treatment should therefore be offered. All health decision-makers must welcome the prospect of a much more focused source of advice and judgement about the effectiveness of different treatments, but NICE leaves us a long way from resolving most of our dilemmas. First, it brings no specific additional or earmarked money with it; and second, it covers only a fraction of the services and treatments which should be offered within the NHS. The result of this inevitable selectivity means that conditions which are *not* the subject of consideration by NICE – or of service standards specified in National Service Frameworks, for instance – may well be left out in the cold when it comes to dividing up the funding cake. It will therefore still be up to the decision-makers to ensure that those services which are not in the spotlight have their day in court.

The way forward

In the light of all this complexity, how can health decision-makers go about trying to achieve legitimacy in their decision-making? An approach which consists of the following principles may help:

- a consistent climate of openness
- a track record of listening
- systematic processes
- explicit values.

Climate of openness

The complex organisational structure of the NHS, to say nothing of the frequent reorganisations, makes openness difficult for the simple reason that the public are not, in general, familiar with the institutions that make decisions on their behalf. It is far easier for the public to recognise doctors, nurses, hospitals and health centres; health authorities and primary care trusts (PCTs) may well be unknown to them or, at best, represent ranks of unnecessary bureaucrats. The fact that clinical staff will play a strong role in PCTs brings a new factor into this equation, and it will be interesting to see whether the public find it any easier to accept GPs and other community practitioners making life-and-death decisions as opposed to the customary *bêtes noires* in grey suits.

This principle of openness raises the further question of whether all papers, without exception, should be made publicly available during the course of the decision-making process. Certainly, the Freedom of Information Act has taken us further in that direction than ever before and it is right that there should be a pre-supposition that information should be shared openly unless there is a defensible reason for it to be withheld. For example, is it acceptable to argue that the need for Boards to think radically and explore the most extreme options provides justification for keeping discussion documents secret – particularly at an early stage of debate? Would the exposure of radical options – many of which might subsequently be discarded – fuel unnecessary concern among the public, let alone a feeding frenzy among the media? Most health decision-makers would argue that such radical thinking should be done in private, but there are two pre-requisites. First, there is a fine judgement to be made between doing initial thinking on the options and discarding the non-runners before going public, and going so far that only a *fait accompli* is served up. Second, it is worth remembering that the public and staff may, if the climate is right, be amongst the most radical thinkers who can genuinely contribute to the debate.

Track record of listening

The second principle is to establish a track record of listening and try to get behind the heat of the moment to understand the real issues. It is easy for positions to become entrenched on the basis of the outward manifestation of a problem rather than on the underlying cause. A number of the examples quoted earlier, such as the isolated paediatric surgery service or specialist work carried out by generalists, may simply appear to local people as a high-handed and careless attempt by bureaucrats to centralise services in a way that is more convenient for staff or managers. It is probably inevitable that such arguments may be presented rather simplistically in the media, but it is essential for health decision-makers to try to address the underlying issue of providing as wide a range of services as possible locally and to achieve real expansion in community and primary care facilities. Such an approach will not make the opposition disappear or quell all fears, but might well offer some reassurance that the local concerns have been genuinely heard and understood.

Communication with the public and evidence of listening does not come quickly, easily or cheaply. At the very least, it will take many hours of people's time, often in the evening and often needing great patience as other items are dealt with on parish council agendas, the Area Forum or the Council Scrutiny Committee. For example, the experience of Avon Health Authority in undertaking an intensive and prolonged period of consultation under the heading 'Choices for Health' was that the opportunity for exchanging views and information by a wide range of community groups and at specially convened meetings was appreciated, and made a genuine contribution to public understanding and exposure of the issues. The vast majority of discussions, however, included at least one contributor declaring: 'Don't ask me to advise on these choices! The more I understand the more awful your job looks. I don't envy you; I don't know how you manage to sleep at night!'

In many areas, the consultation on the establishment of PCTs has reached out into local communities and the new PCTs are expressing a genuine commitment to establish relationships with their local populations so that services can be as locally sensitive and appropriate as possible. Many have already decided to co-opt lay people onto their Boards, and this may be further developed in legislation which brings in new forms of patient representation. The PCTs will labour with a massive agenda in their early months, but it is essential that they continue to give priority to developing this relationship and establishing their identity and bona fides with the population.

Relationships with the media are obviously another part of health decision-makers' communication with the people they serve, and may be only partially susceptible to proactive management. Whilst news editors and reporters – not to mention sub-editors with a predilection for the eye-grabbing headline – will substantially serve their own agenda, honesty, openness and a proactive approach from health decision-makers will at least help to establish relationships on as positive a footing as possible.

Systematic processes

If the processes by which decisions have been made are perceived to have been improper or inadequate, then at worst judicial review might be sought by the aggrieved party. In these circumstances it is essential that health decision-makers can demonstrate the basis on which the decision has been made, taking into account not only the good practice in consultation described above, but also the formal processes adopted by the statutory body, be that a health authority, PCT or NHS trust. Many health authorities in recent years have developed an explicit and comprehensive statement which sets out the authority's decision-making processes, and PCTs are generally adopting a similar approach as they become increasingly responsible for commissioning services. To be relevant, such a statement needs to be debated and adopted in the public meeting of the authority, promulgated widely, reviewed regularly, and followed in practice.

Explicit values

Even with a formal statement of decision-making processes and after the most vigorous programme of engaging with community interests, health decision-makers will still be left with real dilemmas to resolve. The evidence from research and development, the requirements of training programmes, the wishes of staff and even the policies of the Government may continue to be at odds with the wishes of the public. Health decision-makers need to demonstrate that they have taken account honestly, and as fully as possible, of all of these considerations and have weighed them as part of the decision-making process. The final stage in that process should be the application of the values which the organisation has explicitly adopted, referring to such factors as equity, efficiency, responsiveness, accountability, openness and probity. Applying these values will still not make the decision unequivocal or even easy, but they are a crucial part of the debate in which the decision-makers must engage.

If health decision-makers can demonstrate that they have listened and engaged with the public, that they have a formal and rigorous process for decision-making, based on explicit values, not only should they be able to withstand the scrutiny of judicial review, but they should be able to look their population in the eye and sleep in their beds at night.

Chapter 7

Values, ideology and the language of power

Iona Heath

Few people examine their values explicitly; for most people, most of the time, values are simply assumed. It is at times of crisis, both of confidence and morale, that values move more into the foreground, to be scrutinised and either reaffirmed or discarded. It is no coincidence that, over recent years, health care professionals have been preoccupied with values.

The nature of values

A value is an idea: a statement of what is desirable or ought to be, of what is important to the person who holds it. Individual human beings hold an enormous number of different values in hugely various combinations, ranked in different hierarchies that may change over time. This complex abundance of ideas and values is part of what it is to be human:

> We are urged to look upon life as affording a plurality of values, equally genuine, equally ultimate, above all equally objective; incapable, therefore, of being ordered in a timeless hierarchy, or judged in terms of some one absolute standard.[1]

Some values are incompatible, and Isaiah Berlin reminds us that choice is inevitable:

> The notion of the perfect whole, the ultimate solution, in which all good things coexist, seems to me to be not merely unattainable – that is a truism – but conceptually incoherent; I do not know what is meant by a harmony of this kind. Some among the Great Goods cannot live together. That is a conceptual truth. We are doomed to choose, and every choice may entail an irreparable loss.[2]

We inherit values from our parents and take on those of our peers or people, both real and fictional, who we admire, and we hone and refine our values across a lifetime. Children learn values both explicitly through our teaching and implicitly through the ways in which we choose to live our lives. Each of us reconsiders and reorders our values according to the circumstances of our lives and we are all forced into a range of compromises. Our values drive our sense of right and wrong, our notion of the good. They represent our aspirations, our hopes for our lives and for those of others. They provide 'an orientation, which is not merely a sense of direction, but a sense of where the centre of the world is and how to get there'.[3] Inevitably, the values to which we aspire are not always fulfilled in the decisions we make in the messy reality of daily life. This gap between aspiration and reality drives both motivation and guilt, and the challenge is always to close the gap – to strive, with W B Yeats:

> *to hold in a single thought reality and justice.*[4]

Some values endure; others come and go. Some have quite staggering longevity and, surviving almost as long as human history, must reflect fundamental aspects of the human condition. Such values include justice, truth and freedom. Others, such as efficiency, effectiveness and quality, are much more recent.

Values are expressed and communicated in language, and for the individual in dialogue with others, language is a subtle and flexible vehicle that goes a long way towards reflecting the complex interactions between different values and ideas. As we find and use words, each of us annexes them to ourselves, imprinting our own understanding and meaning on the words we have chosen. It is this process that keeps language alive, constantly changing and fragmenting. Language is always historical, centred in present usage, but reflecting what we have understood in the past and dictating how we will understand the future:

> *The world is different after it has been read by a Shakespeare or an Emily Dickinson or a Samuel Beckett because it has been augmented by their reading of it.*[5]

Language and values become mutually reinforcing.

Values in health care

The necessary focus of health care is illness, and almost all illness, however apparently trivial, evokes fear. Fear lurks, mostly unexpressed, within the symptoms of illness, and the fear may be of the disruption of career, of interference with an important life event, of implications for other family members, of a specific diagnosis which holds particular dread, of pain, of serious chronic disease or disability, of life never being the same again, and, ultimately, of untimely death. Fear runs through all the transactions of health care and, to a great extent, dictates the values of those directly involved. Throughout history, values in health care have been concerned with the very particular vulnerability of those who are ill and the protection and dignity that they are owed.

Fear makes us feel vulnerable, and fear which proves unfounded makes us feel foolish. Fear can only be held and addressed by trust. Any health care professional who has been seriously ill and frightened will know that knowledge is not enough:

> *Because it can only be shared,*
> *like a waltz*
> *or trust.*[6]

Trust develops between individuals. The basic unit of health care is the consultation within which a person who is ill, or believes himself or herself to be ill, seeks the advice of a trusted other.[7] By tradition, health care professionals have been selected and educated, with varying degrees of success, to uphold values which foster trust, such as confidentiality, consent, integrity, personal commitment and continuity of care. Similarly, any abuse of trust is viewed as deeply reprehensible.

Illness happens to unique individuals who hold values of their own. The language of health care needs to find ways of accommodating the values of each vulnerable individual and give expression to the vocational values of health care professionals. Per Fugelli has described medicine as:

> *biology* × *individuality* × *politics squared.*[8]

And again, each of these aspects evokes values which have a place within the language of health care.

The transition from values to ideology

An ideology is broader than a value and indicates a systematic scheme of ideas relating to the conduct of a group or society. Individuals hold values; at the level of society, values become ideology.

The transition from values to ideology is hazardous. Individuals hold hugely varied combinations of values and much is lost when this rich resource is constrained into an ideology. The process is inevitably political and shaped by the interests of dominant groups, wherever they appear on the political spectrum. Values are chosen because they support a preferred view or course of action. Too often the resulting ideology represents a fiction – 'those arrangements which are offered as truth by power's window-dressers everywhere'[9] – and the intention is to control. Values may be subverted by the politics of ideology and, in the process, the aspirations of individuals are either bolstered or lost:

> *He had been driven from the paradise of simple faith in Emperor and Virtue, Truth, and Justice, and, now fettered in silence and endurance, he may have realized that the stability of the world, the power of laws, and the glory of majesties were all based on deviousness.*[10]

Like values, ideology finds expression in language. At the level of the individual, language is centrifugal, changed by each usage and infinitely adaptable to human aspiration:

> *The word, directed towards its object, enters a dialogically agitated and tension-filled environment of alien words, value judgments and accents, weaves in and out of complex interrelationships, merges with some, recoils from others, intersects with yet a third group …*[11]

Or, described metaphorically:

> *A game of Chinese whispers. A hot word thrown into the next lap before it burns. It has not been allowed to set. Each hand that momentarily holds it, weighs it, before depositing it with a neighbour also, inadvertently, moulds it; communicates its own heat.*[12]

However, at the level of society and ideology, language becomes fixed, normative and centripetal. Dialogue is replaced by iteration and, eventually, convergence in the interests of the powerful:

> *The language expresses the ideology, and conveys it, imprints it on our minds, and moulds our attitudes, our ethics.*[13]

This convergent language of ideology rapidly becomes degraded, losing much of the flexibility of the language of individual values:

> As soon as certain topics are raised, the concrete melts into the abstract and no one seems able to think in turns of speech that are not hackneyed: prose consists less and less of words chosen for the sake of their meaning, and more and more of phrases tacked together like the sections of a prefabricated henhouse.[14]

How easily Orwell would have recognised the reincarnation of double-speak as 'spin'. He understood exactly how language, used in this way, performs the important service of concealing meaning even from the speaker.

Ideologies have power to unite or to divide communities. History shows us very clearly that the ideology of a majority poses real threats to any readily identifiable minority. Within a dominant ideology, it becomes very easy for the values of minorities to be marginalised and even ridiculed, and the more vulnerable the minority, the greater the threat. Nevertheless, it is an ideology that drives the behaviour of a social institution, and without a coherent system of values, amounting to an ideology, there is a danger that social institutions become incapable of consistent functioning. At all levels of social organisation, from family to nation state, ideology is both an asset and a danger. Perhaps the best outcome is the retention of as broad a range of values as possible, combined with choices which are transitory and negotiable. Such 'a humanistic, multi-valued conception of public rationality'[15] allows the accommodation of a proportionately greater measure of individual aspiration and is thereby inclusive and enabling.

The National Health Service

In the United Kingdom, the National Health Service has been the dominant social institution for more than half a century. It was the immediate product of the apparently unprecedented social solidarity that arose out of the experience of the Second World War, and, from its inception, the NHS was designed to be inclusive, funded from general taxation to provide health care for all citizens on the basis of need.[16] In this way, the NHS was framed as a risk-sharing social contract, created by all citizens for all citizens and essentially dependent on the democratic assumption of equal rights for all.

> The nature of our society is strongly reflected in the values embodied in national health care arrangements; transactions involved in health care delivery are the main way these values are experienced; given the significance

of health in everyday life, these transactions are therefore an important part of the way our sense of society is constituted.[17]

The founding ideology of the Health Service was one of universality and social justice – democratic governance being used deliberately by an avowedly socialist administration to protect the needs of the poor and vulnerable. The most immediate task of the NHS was the expert care of sick people and this gave wide scope for the flourishing of professional values. Professional judgement and expertise were prioritised at the expense of patient choice and autonomy.

The rise of public health introduced an alternative ideology. The care of individuals and the care of populations dictate different priorities and evoke different values. In public health, the imperative to seek the greatest good for the greatest number promotes utilitarian values such as effectiveness and efficiency, which are prioritised at the expense of the professional commitment to the continuing care of the sick individual. Public health seeks to rank the needs of different groups of individuals. Clinical professionals find such ranking almost unbearably problematic.

In the 1980s, in the wake of the global demise of communism and the consequently uncontested rise of global capitalism, government 'reform' of the NHS introduced the ideology of the market and yet another competing set of values. Efficiency, competition and the notion of the patient as a self-interested consumer, were all prioritised. The incompatibility of conflicting value systems seemed to reach a critical point, and demoralised clinical professionals felt that their commitment to the care of individual patients was being systematically undervalued.

Postmodernism generated a distrust of the comprehensive explanations, the destabilisation of many existing values and ideologies, and further erosion of the implicit monopolies of professional knowledge and expertise.

Postmodernism is self-consciously pluralistic and multicultural, a freewheeling consortium of heterogeneous parts, where underlying consistencies are often less visible than the outward play of difference.[18]

Simultaneously, the widespread collapse of religious belief has driven an apparent desire to prolong life indefinitely, whatever the cost in both human and financial terms; a desire which is enthusiastically fuelled by the pharmaceutical and health technology industries. The perennial human pursuit of utopia has shifted from a search for the perfect human society to the increasingly desperate quest for the perfect solitary human body.

The rhetoric of health care has reflected these ideological shifts, and the NHS as a social institution has sought to retain all these incompatible value systems within its creaking frame. Remarkably, despite the disintegration of social solidarity and the decline of postwar socialist values, the fundamental social contract to provide health care for all remains intact, with the single exception of the frail elderly. The irony is that the social contract can only be enacted within relationships of trust between individuals.

The necessary focus of health care must always be on the needs of each unique individual, whose particular life history dictates his or her own values and priorities. This focus engenders a robust awareness of, and defence against, the limitations of ideology. When the ideology driving the Service becomes too simplistic, the limitations become obvious to both patients and clinical professionals, but – and here is the political danger – only to the minority of patients who are actively engaged in the health care system at any one time.

> *We should be on our guard against the ease with which simplified models tend to take over and look like the whole of reality. We should resist that tendency.*[15]

Simple systems have no place for uncertainty and yet almost all the transactions of health care are about degrees of uncertainty. The plurality of values accommodated within the NHS will always be both its greatest strength and a significant weakness. Successive governments yearn for a standardised technical service delivering units of high-quality health care, but a standardised service is appropriate only to standardised patients with standardised illnesses. There is no standard unit of either fear or trust.

Who gains and who loses from particular models of health care delivery? The aspirations of the powerful dictate which values and therefore which evidence and which facts are prioritised. Over the last 50 years we have seen the gradual waning of professional power, displaced by the waxing of the power of private capital, exemplified most recently by New Labour's enthusiastic espousal of private–public partnership and stubborn support for the continuation of Private Finance Initiatives. It is no coincidence that, since the market revolution of the 1980s, we have lost the explicit public ownership that provided the risk-sharing foundation of the NHS. It has been recast in a series of risk averse institutions – the ever-permutating panoply of trusts and authorities, each with its own independent finances and driven by the requirement to balance the books.

The language of health care has changed almost beyond recognition. Cost-effectiveness has become the pre-eminent virtue. Failures of health have been blamed on the lifestyles of individuals, and failures of treatment on the incompetence of professionals. Throughout this period, the NHS has become less and less democratically accountable. Between 1948 and 1974, local authority health departments were part of the structure of the NHS[19] and, until the 'reforms' of the 1980s, local authorities were still represented on the boards of health authorities. Now the fragmented governance of a multitude of NHS institutions is almost entirely appointed and the opportunity to restore even the most tokenistic degree of local accountability has not been taken. It is increasingly obvious that a democratic deficit in public services favours the interests of multinational corporations.[20] Health care companies and property developers are able to expand into the ownership and provision of health care premises, unimpeded by processes of local scrutiny.[21]

Without a democratic framework, the social contract between all citizens for all citizens is seriously weakened. Individuals begin to demand a high level of service for themselves and their families, while declining to support the level of taxation necessary to fund the NHS at such a high level for all. Mutual obligation as a civic duty begins to disappear. However, democracy as an aspirational value, despite its persistence across human history, is not without its conflicts.[22] Powerful local democracy enforces different priorities for different communities and tends to erode equity and generate postcode lotteries of care. Beyond this lurks the ever-present danger that a powerful majority, wielding its democratic muscle, will systematically ignore the needs of vulnerable minorities; a danger which was manifest in the first round of priority setting under the Oregon Health Plan.

Nonetheless, there is evidence to suggest that both social capital and active participatory democracy are actively health-promoting. We begin to understand the processes by which a sense of having little control over one's own life circumstances, and a lack of social affiliations and security, activate biological pathways that link stress and chronic anxiety to observable physiological changes that undermine health.[23] It begins to appear that the founding values of the NHS – universality and democracy – have the capacity not only to treat but also to prevent illness.

Alternatives to ideology

... the richer our scheme of values, the harder it will prove to effect harmony within it. The more open we are to the presence of value, of divinity, in the world, the more surely conflict closes us in. The price of harmonization seems to be impoverishment, the price of richness disharmony.[24]

If the NHS is to remain inclusive, ideology may be a damaging means of perpetuating values, because it cedes the language and ranking of values to the powerful. Story, myth and metaphor have a much greater capacity for complexity and uncertainty and for reflecting a wider diversity of values. As the present Government has discovered to its cost, 'cradle to grave' is one example of a myth that has gained a very strong grip on the popular imagination. The phrase has come to express many people's understanding of the implications of social justice and their expectations of the Health Service. The desperate assertion that such a promise was never made has done nothing to undermine its force.

Using qualitative techniques, both patients and citizens could be purposefully selected to provide diverse stories which express both their direct experience and expectations of the health service and their hopes for it. In this way, it might be possible to construct a credible democracy of ideas and values, but only if the politically and professionally powerful can be restrained from editing the contributions of those who are less often heard. This could be combined with ensuring that all decisions are much more transparent and designing overt mechanisms for ensuring that many more voices are heard in the debate, particularly those of the vulnerable and socially excluded. Democratic 'outreach' initiatives might even extend to obliging people to participate in certain democratic activities, as part of the delivery of care, enabling genuine influence far exceeding the current charade of public consultation and patient satisfaction surveys. Such initiatives could serve to enrich the values that underpin the NHS and offer ways of uniting a huge and diverse service in the common endeavour of providing care for each one of us.

References

1   Berlin I. Alleged relativism in eighteenth-century European thought. In: *The Crooked Timber of Humanity*. London: Fontana Press, 1990.
2   Berlin I. The pursuit of the ideal. In: *The Crooked Timber of Humanity*. London: Fontana Press, 1990.

3   Toon P. *Towards a Philosophy of General Practice: a study of the virtuous practitioner.* Occasional Paper 78. Exeter: Royal College of General Practitioners, 1999.

4   Yeats W B. *A Vision.* London: Macmillan, 1962.

5   Heaney S. Joy or night. In: *The Redress of Poetry: Oxford lectures.* London: Faber and Faber, 1995.

6   Burnside J. Flora. *The Guardian* 2001; 13 January.

7   Spence J. *The Purpose and Practice of Medicine.* Oxford: Oxford University Press, 1960.

8   Fugelli P. Rød resept. Essays om perfeksjon, prestasjon og helse. Oslo: Tano Aschehoug, 1999.

9   Heaney S. The atlas of civilization. In: *The Government of the Tongue.* London: Faber and Faber, 1988.

10 Roth J. *The Radetsky March.* London: Penguin, 1995.

11 Bakhtin M M. *The Dialogic Imagination: four essays.* Austin: University of Texas Press, 1981.

12 Cook E. *Achilles.* London: Methuen Publishing Ltd, 2001.

13 Dunstan G R. *Ideology, Ethics and Practice.* London: RCGP, 1994.

14 Orwell G. Politics and the English language. In: *The Collected Essays, Journalism and Letters of George Orwell. Volume 4. In Front of Your Nose, 1945–1950.* London: Secker & Warburg, 1968.

15 Nussbaum M C. *Poetic Justice: the literary imagination and public life.* Boston, Massachusetts: Beacon Press, 1995.

16 Ministry of Health. *A National Health Service.* Cmd. 6502. London: HMSO, 1944.

17 Towell D. Revaluing the NHS: empowering ourselves to shape a health care system fit for the 21st century. *Policy and Politics* 1996; 24 (3): 287–97.

18 Morris D B. *Illness and Culture in the Postmodern Age.* Berkeley: University of California Press, 1998: 24.

19 Watkins S J. For debate: public health 2020. *BMJ* 1994; 309: 1147–9.

20 Price D, Pollock A M, Shaoul J. How the World Trade Organisation is shaping domestic policies in health care. *Lancet* 1999; 354: 1889–92.

21 Pollock A M, Player S, Godden S. How private finance is moving primary care into corporate ownership. *BMJ* 2001; 322: 960–3.

22 New B. *A Good-Enough Service: values, trade-offs and the NHS.* London: Institute for Public Policy Research and King's Fund, 1999.

23 Wilkinson R. *Mind the Gap – hierarchies, health and human evolution.* London: Weidenfeld & Nicolson, 2000.

24 Nussbaum M C. *The Fragility of Goodness. Luck and Ethics in Greek Tragedy and Philosophy.* Cambridge: Cambridge University Press, 1986.

Chapter 8

Healing the multiple wounds: medicine in a multicultural society

Ziauddin Sardar

The model of the NHS as a publicly funded health service free at the point of use for all citizens is claimed to be the UK's gift to the modern civilised world. However, from the perspective of a multicultural UK in the twenty-first century there is a problem with this statement. This is not related to issues of under-funding, the crumbling of infrastructure, postcode lotteries, privatisation by overt or covert policy, or the ethical dilemmas and exponentially increasing costs of high-tech medicine. The problem is one of provenance and therefore the universality of values invoked in support of the National Health Service.

The first public hospital dispensing treatment freely at the point of need to any citizen opened its doors in Baghdad in 809AD, a fact that British Muslims should be quick and insistent in pointing out. Soon, no Muslim city was without the kind of hospital we are familiar with today, with specialist wards where patients were assigned according to their ailment and treatment needs. The hospitals were organised as teaching institutions where medical and pharmacological education and qualifications were standardised and regulated by state authorities. They were centres of excellence for the advancement of clinical understanding where medical and surgical practice was pioneered.[1] Although supported by state funds, the hospitals also received funding from one of the most ubiquitous institutions in Muslim history, *waqfs* – private charitable foundations and endowments made in perpetuity for designated usage, provision of health care being prominent along with education.

How Baghdad, the newly created city soon to be the capital of the Abbasid Caliphate, came to have free public hospitals is neither a mystery nor a quirk of history. It was the logical outcome of basic Islamic values which, at that precise moment in history, were being crystallised and institutionalised in Muslim consciousness and social practice. Provision for the infirm, the sick and the needy is one of the functions for which *zakat*, the annual welfare obligation often translated as the 'poor tax' and described as one of the five pillars of

Islam, is paid by all Muslims according to their financial means. The State used zakat and other sources of funds, such as waqfs, to set up a network of hospitals; a national health service established long before the creation of the National Health Service in the UK.

Free medical treatment for all at the point of need is a core Islamic value. Making this point is not a 'me first' piece of one-upmanship, it is a reminder of how narrow the focus usually is in the public debate of what are termed 'universal' values. To look at the universe solely from the perspective of British or Western history is restrictive and limiting. The UK's Health Service is an expression of core Western values as they came to be understood and institutionalised at a particular point in history. But it is not only an expression of Western values; it involves the values of many other cultures and civilisations, just as these have found institutionalised expression in other histories. If this is not acknowledged, we inevitably ignore the wider, universal foundations on which we must build to achieve shared values in a multicultural society.

Values are derived from the world-view by and through which we live. How we enjoy life, what we think of our bodies, how we treat them and how we shape our environment, are all governed by our world-view. While world-views shape lifestyle, our lifestyles determine our health status. In his highly regarded *Diseases of Civilization*,[2] Brian Inglis lists heart disease, cancer, mental illness, infectious diseases and iatrogenic disorders (illnesses induced by doctors and their treatments) as the main illnesses of Western civilisation. With the exception of iatrogenic disorders, all the illnesses are related to lifestyle. For example, heart disease is a consequence of affluence, the result of overeating, rich food, refined foods, stress, chemicals in the environment and lack of physical exercise. Lifestyles not only produce new illnesses: they can also radically transform existing diseases. These can be reactivated, or assume newer deadly forms. For example, in the early nineteenth century, polio existed in the USA as a mild childhood illness. It started to disappear in the 1920s as US cities began to clean and purify their water supplies. However, a few decades later it came back, and this time it had the potential to kill and cripple. It had now become a disease of affluence, the consequence of pure drinking water. Consider also herpes, which has been with us in a harmless form for centuries as cold sores. As genital herpes it assumes a newer, more irritating form: sexual behaviour has changed the epidemiology of the disease. World-views not only shape lifestyles; they also affect the external environment in which we live. This plays just as important a role in producing diseases as lifestyles themselves. Many modern health problems can be linked to environmental factors. For example, the rise of infertility amongst men in the USA has been traced to toxins like PCBs, which concentrate in men's reproductive organs, drastically reducing sperm counts. Over the last half century, the sperm counts of Western men have decreased by 50 per cent, the size of the male organ has shrunk, and the incidence of malformed penises, undescended testes and other reproductive disorders has increased.

There is, therefore, a close relationship between world-views and health. By promoting certain lifestyles and producing an environment in which these can flourish, world-views determine the state of health of individuals and societies. They also form the matrix within which attempts are made to find cures for illnesses and promote health. Medicine is equally linked to world-views. Modern medicine is a product of the world-view of Western civilisation. and non-Western medical systems – Islamic, Chinese, Ayurvedic – are products of their respective civilisations and world-views.[3]

A multicultural society, by definition, contains a number of distinct groups with a diversity of world-views. Identifying the points of convergence, the common principles and shared values of different world-views is a necessary step in uncovering the creative strength of a genuine multicultural society. The idea that UK institutions might benefit from the values of other cultures, those of the migrant populations now part of society, is a kind of multiculturalism we have not yet conceived. But without incorporating certain values and approaches to medicine from other world-views in our public and health policies, we cannot achieve any meaningful multiculturalism.

An inclusive approach could be thought of in paternalist terms, as some kind of benevolent nod to migrant culture, but the exercise has to be carried out for the benefit of the UK as a whole. In a multicultural society that was confident, informed and alert, shared values and common principles would provide renewed strength and resilience for basic institutions like the Health Service. Such a society would be able to develop a more creative dialogue of values and explore new insights and ways of thinking by looking at familiar arguments from a new perspective. Although shared principles do exist, different cultures and world-views have distinctive ways of building these principles into social patterns and structures of argument. Common values and shared principles can mean much more than platitudes or simplistic truisms; they can help us see the many ways in which values can be made relevant and given a practical form in new kinds of delivery systems, such as patient empowerment, doctor–patient relationships and community care.

The greatest impediment to incorporating non-Western values in the National Health Service is that other world-views are not considered to be equal within UK society. This is reflected in the language of inferiority used to describe non-Western medicines as 'alternative', 'complementary' and 'traditional' systems. Such terminology not only equates a sophisticated and socially objective system of medicine such as the Chinese with more recent New Age upstarts, it also relegates them to a substandard position by definition.

The first step towards accommodating the non-Western world-views that continue to influence the social habits and ways of life of minority groups within modern UK society must be to look at medicine itself in a radically different way. It is already acknowledged that multiculturalism is changing medicine in a practical sense. For example, we now see the epidemiology of a multicultural society as a new challenge: the incidence of heart disease and diabetes are much higher among Pakistani and Bangladeshi populations, sickle cell anaemia affects Afro-Caribbean and African Britons. Gradually, it has been recognised that non-Western ideas and attitudes must be respected, both as a matter of basic principle and civil right, and to ensure the effective delivery of rights and services to minority groups. As a result, we have health workers with appropriate language skills and knowledge of different cultural practices, there is access to and increased numbers of female doctors and, through work with the broad range of community groups and organisations, the use of available health services is being encouraged. Accommodation of difference is an important aspect of achieving social inclusion, and a significant value in our multicultural society. However, the multiculturalism of pragmatism and difference is a long way from engaging with other world-views as equal partners in a dialogue of values.

Constructing a dialogue of values requires seeing medicine in a totally different light. Our popular, common-sense understanding of the term is exclusively of modern Western medicine.[4] This is a myopic, ahistorical view, one that assumes there was nothing before the arrival of modern medicine, that diseases, sickness, ill health and premature death were the norm before the emergence of the modern scientific miracle. It suggests that nothing that existed before modern medicine is really important since it has been completely superseded. What we now know envelopes all the past, making it irrelevant and incapable of making any significant contribution to the concept or practice of modern medicine. So prevalent is this view that we can no longer imagine what it was like not to know what is now common knowledge among the expert adepts, the specialists and professionals. It is therefore necessary to remind ourselves that what we call modern medicine is 60 years old, and began with the development of penicillin. Until 120 years ago, when Pasteur pioneered the germ theory of disease, Western medicine was not only like medicine in all other civilisations, it was in large measure a product of knowledge and expertise acquired from other cultures. Only the advent of penicillin and antibiotics transformed medicine from a healing art into a true science in the mechanistic mould constructed as the idealised view of Western science. The great and very recent leap forward is supposedly epitomised by the defeat of the great epidemic diseases, most notably the eradication of smallpox. This vision of history is now a distinct tradition that underlines the separation of the West from its own history and the incommensurability of modern Western values with those of all other civilisations.

The rewriting of history eradicates how much the present competence and expertise of modern medicine owes to non-Western civilisations. For example, the medical encyclopaedia of Abu al-Qasim al-Zahrawi (c. 936–1013) illustrated the basic set of surgical instruments that would be recognised by modern surgeons. Known in European history as 'Albucasis', his book was available long before its contents became incorporated into the normal practice of surgery in Europe. What we now denigratingly describe as 'alternative' or 'complementary' medicine was in fact the foundation on which modern medicine is built. It also hides the degree to which new developments in medicine are being affected by appropriating, without attribution, knowledge from traditional non-Western medicines – ethno-pharmacology and its scramble to patent new drugs being a notable example. This rewriting of history traps us in an inherently monocultural outlook, and makes conceiving a genuine multiculturalism almost impossible. It makes it difficult to acknowledge that, until the arrival of penicillin, Western medicine was essentially the same as Islamic medicine. In both cultures, Ibn Sina's (980–1037) *Canons of Medicine* was a standard text for centuries. In 1716, Lady Mary Wortley Montagu, wife of the British Ambassador to the Ottoman court in Istanbul, became fascinated by the widely practised technique of infecting healthy people with a weakened strain of smallpox to give immunity. Lady Wortley Montagu took a keen interest because she herself was badly scarred by smallpox, a common enough occurrence in Europe at that time. On her return to Britain, she popularised the technique among the social elite. Before that, al-Razi (854–935), the renowned Muslim doctor and scientist, had described the disease in such detail that his observations are considered a scientific marvel even today.[5] Yet, Western medicine confers the pioneering breakthrough, the invention of a smallpox vaccine, to Edward Jenner (1749–1823), and the victory over smallpox to the medical delivery systems of the twentieth century.

My argument is that Western medicine should be seen not as something apart from history, but as a tradition. Indeed, it is the youngest of a number of great traditions of medicine. It is not *the* medicine, the standard absolute, but a way of practising medicine within a world-view. When scientific medicine first appeared it was thought to have miraculous powers and a death-defying capacity. It is little wonder that ordinary people were filled with awe at its potential. Modern medicine has a right to be arrogant, I would concede, but it also has the responsibility and the obligation to regard itself as a tradition and submit itself to the associated discipline.

Tradition is not a given. It is, in an ideal sense at least, negotiated and contested. It provides a context for debate, allowing testing, tempering and amelioration, subject to an enduring set of values, ethical constraints and overriding purposes to promote enhancement by both change and continuity. Viewing Western medicine as a tradition, we not only bring its values, constraints and moral and ethical parameters to the fore, but also imagine how it can grow beyond its narrow confines and transcend the dilemmas it encounters or creates. When we see medicine in this way it allows us to debate the balance between healing and disease eradication, and all the attendant questions that arise. Moreover, it becomes possible to see other traditions of medicine as equally valid, and to highlight the similarities between traditions as well as critically evaluate their differences. But if medicine remains an absolute, detached from history and a non-tradition, such debates and the new lines of enquiry they could promote are impossible, and a genuine multicultural discourse of values becomes a utopian pipedream.

From the non-Western perspective, two values in particular are important. The first is context. Non-Western traditions of medicine place a great deal of emphasis on the context of the patient, with family, social and financial circumstances important factors in diagnosis. Modern medicine sees the human body as a machine made up of a number of different parts – the organs. Diseases are well-defined entities responsible for structural changes in the cells of the body and tend to have singular causes. They are caused by germs, bacteria and viruses; recently it has been accepted – only in the face of mounting evidence – that environment too is a causative agent. The body is attacked by outside forces and if these external factors are isolated and crushed, by chemical or surgical intervention, the body can be repaired and the patient cured. In contrast, non-Western medical systems look at the body in holistic terms. Illness can be caused as much by personal, social and environmental circumstances as by disease.

The point is not that the Western, reductive mechanistic approach should be abandoned, but that context should be integrated into the way we think about sickness and health. We need to do that not only because the reductive model, despite the propaganda on its behalf, has been successful in only a few special cases, such as acute infectious processes, but also because it cannot explain the overwhelming majority of illnesses. Nor is this approach to medicine responsible for the immense improvements in human health and lifespan. The decline of the mortality rate over the past century owes almost nothing to modern medicine. The credit belongs, as recent research has shown, to pure or treated drinking water, pasteurised milk, indoor plumbing, closed sewers, improved nutrition, clean and safe workplaces and shorter working hours. In other words, improvements in health came through improvements in social context. As Thomas McKeown has shown in his elaborate historical-epidemiological studies, modern medicine cured individuals but had little impact in the overall improvement of health in industrialised Europe in the late nineteenth century.[6] After examining the possible causes for declining mortality, he finally settled for improved nutrition. A similar study in the USA attributed the fall in mortality rates to the disappearance of 11 major diseases: influenza, whooping cough, polio, typhoid, smallpox, scarlet fever, measles, diphtheria, tuberculosis, pneumonia and problems of the digestive system.[7] With the exception of the first three, all the other diseases had died out almost entirely before the advent of medical intervention. So, our own research and experience shows that broader context is important.

In non-Western traditions of medicine, the first question is why an illness occurs, and the diagnosis aims at removing the conditions that lead to it. Modern medicine tries to understand the biological mechanism through which the disease operates, thus curing the individual but leaving the conditions that produce the illness intact. Thus, on the question of the rise in infertility amongst US men, emphasis is not placed on removing the toxins in the environment which cause infertility. Instead, enormous financial and intellectual resources have been expended on finding ways and means of making infertile men fertile again. Further valuable resources have been devoted to the collateral approach: developing the whole technology of artificial insemination by donors to allow women, either as individuals or as part of an infertile couple, to bypass the entire problem. A more balanced approach requires bringing the wider context back into medicine.

The second non-Western value relates to power. In non-Western traditions of medicine, the power of healing belongs to patients and not doctors. Ultimately, doctors can offer remedies but they work with the power of the patient. In Western medicine, the patient is not only totally helpless but society itself is removed from medicine. If disease and illness are external to the body, and sickness is cured by isolating the disease and exterminating it, then the role of society in both producing and treating sickness becomes irrelevant. By trying to simultaneously identify and manage ill health and conceal its origins – the entrenchment of health and illness in social and economic relations – modern medicine operates as an ideologically constructed power structure. The power of the medical establishment, the consultants and the doctors, is absolute. No wonder patients arriving in a hospital perceive themselves as helpless victims whose only function is to bring diseases for the doctors to fight and defeat. As a result, an expectant mother, as I discovered during the birth of my own children, becomes a helpless patient who is 'ill'. Pregnancy is not seen as a natural condition but as a form of sickness that can only be cured in hospital. A world-view that places no premium on family life, indeed actively undermines family relations, is bound to see the home as an unsafe place to give birth. In the UK, it is against the law to practise childbirth at home, unattended by qualified medical practitioners. And doctors who encourage natural childbirth are sometimes disciplined. Nature cannot be trusted to produce a normal birth; it has to be actively managed by technology. Even though obstetric procedures often do more harm than good, it is not always obvious to the victim who is led to believe that home births are infinitely more dangerous. The most common danger to women in labour is haemorrhaging, and the remedy involves plasma and sterile water. However, midwives are not allowed these supplies, not because they cannot administer plasma drips but because by handing over even this limited amount of technology the medical establishment would undermine its own control and power.

Childbirth is not the only aspect of natural life that has become medicalised and passed from the control of the individual into the domain of the medical profession. Obesity has become a medical condition, eating and the epidemic spread of eating disorders are medical issues, and depression has become one of the most common ailments and reasons for drug intervention in Western life. If we have not yet made life a full-blown disease, we have certainly expanded the definition and number of treatable conditions beyond the carrying capacity of general practitioners. What has passed into the power and territory of the medical profession cannot emerge unless we adopt a more sustainable view of health as well as disease and medical intervention.

With such a power structure in place, there is little sense in talking about non-Western values or indeed a viable national health service for a multicultural society. In these circumstances, systems of medicine based on other world-views are naturally seen as a threat to the power and domination of modern medicine. On a very simple level, they present an economic threat. In the Western world-view, both health care systems and diseases are commodities. Medicine is about income, and advances in modern medicine are not made with health in mind but for financial rewards, as well as prestige and fame. Witness the history of heart transplants. But beyond economics, non-Western medical systems threaten the notion of modernity itself. That is why, under colonialism, these systems were ruthlessly suppressed, their research centres closed, and their practitioners threatened and in some cases killed. In India, Islamic and Ayurvedic medicine were declared inferior, irrelevant and outlawed.[8] In Tunisia, many *hakims*, practitioners of Islamic medicine, were charged with subverting the State and sentenced to death for practising their art of healing.[9] We need to break this power structure, not just to allow non-Western values and medical systems to be incorporated into the National Health Service but also because such authoritarianism is no longer viable. The recent case of Dr Harold Shipman, who, unsuspected and undetected for decades, mass-murdered his patients, and that of consultant gynaecologist Rodney Ledward, whose botched operations over 16 years maimed more than 400 women, well illustrate the deficiencies of the system.

It is the emphasis on the whole person and the power of the patient to heal her/himself that has made non-Western medical systems so popular in the UK. Patients are discovering what this approach can achieve. It delivers cures, relief of symptoms and a quality of caring for the patient as a whole person that has slipped out of the practice of modern medicine. Its cures, therapies and medications have developed and evolved over very long periods of time and have extensive experimental and anecdotal evidence to support their efficacy. The form in which this wealth of evidence is preserved may not always appear commensurate with modern scientific practice, but this only takes us back to the idea of world-views and the embedded nature of theories and evidence within them. What most UK users of non-Western medical systems know is that they offer a cure in less potent and invasive ways, having fewer unwelcome or unwanted side effects. That is why increasing numbers of affluent, educated people are choosing traditional therapies, at their own expense, over modern medicine. It is also leading the medical profession to accept the efficacy of some traditional therapies and increasingly to include them within the context of modern medical practice.

But there are other reasons why this shift in emphasis is important. Non-Western therapies can be expensive lifestyle options in Western society. In much of the rest of the world – the Third World where these systems originate and continue to exist – they are cheaper, more easily and more widely available than modern medicine. They meet the expectations and preferences of people in ways modern medicine does not. Non-Western therapies present a basic idea people find easy to accept – that health promotion is a good thing, that it is a long-term proposition, and that it is not the work of medicine alone. The generation brought up on instant gratification has matured into the generation that recognises a basic choice. You can take a pill that can knock you out for a couple of days and cure your illness and symptoms quickly, but with very real possibilities of side effects. Or, a better result can be obtained over a longer period by traditional means that will not make you feel like a zombie in the meantime nor have unpleasant side effects. A further realisation comes with non-Western therapies: the longer you take to deal with the illness the more you learn about yourself, your own body, and the other subtle aids to promoting health that have always been part of this approach to medicine. Paying customers like the idea of empowering themselves to take control of their own health.

If we make the transition from modern scientific medicine as the absolute standard to a tradition of medicine, a distinctive way of thinking and acting, it becomes interlinked with other systems of medicine. Seeing modern medicine as a tradition opens another field of consideration: all traditions can also atrophy and decline, becoming obscurantist and tyrannous, and seeking to dominate instead of uplifting the human condition. We know there are imperfections in both the conception and practice of modern medicine. However, we have acute difficulty in finding ways to debate the problems of a system that often gives the appearance of being a juggernaut careering beyond our ability to re-establish reasoned controls. It is equally true that the traditions of non-Western medicines have atrophied under the onslaught of modernity. Not everything extant as traditional medicine is valuable, noble and positive. Charlatans and quacks are no longer to be found only on the wider fringes of traditional non-Western medicine and 'alternative' therapies; they are also within the domain of scientific medicine. Not all commensurability is positive and idyllic, but the purpose and nature of a living tradition is to provide the means of tackling the bad just as much as promoting the good.

In the end, genuine multiculturalism in medicine, as much as in society as a whole, is not a question of different values. It is more that the complex questions of what medicine should do and how it should do it are approached differently in non-Western systems – and provide us with new ways of finding answers. It may also be that non-Western traditions have retained more of the ideals of healing and health promotion, including environmental health provision, because they have been on the outside, lacking access to modern medicine. These attitudes could provide the ballast modern medicine needs to develop as a more humane tradition. There is more at stake here than bowing to public demand and market forces, whose place in medicine I would vigorously question, whether modern or non-Western. And there is definitely more involved than simply a grudging acknowledgement of the fact that non-Western medical systems work. There is a problem of definition that we need the honesty to acknowledge. The recent resurgence of non-Western medicine and traditional therapies point to philosophical lacunae in the concept and practice of modern medicine – its failure to develop as a tradition and therefore to mature beyond the arrogance of adolescence into the humility and wisdom of age. As traditions, the diversity of systems of medicine can learn from each other, interact and co-operate with each other. Medicine then becomes a model of how a multicultural society operates, as an ongoing dialogue of values among citizens sharing equal responsibility for improving the well-being of society as a whole.

References

1   Dols M W. The origins of the Islamic hospital: myth and reality. *Bulletin of History of Medicine* 1987; 61: 367–90.
2   Inglis B. *Diseases of Civilization*. London: Paladin, 1981.
3   For a more detailed discussion of world-views and medicine, see Sardar Z. Medicine and metaphysics. In: Sardar Z, editor. *The Revenge of Athena: science, exploitation and the Third World*. London: Mansell, 1988.
4   Just as we see modern science as *the* science, the only systematic and objective way to study nature. See Sardar Z. Above, beyond and at the centre of science wars: a postcolonial reading. In: Ashman K, Baringer P, editors. *After the Science Wars*.

London: Routledge, 2001: 120–39.

5   For a general introduction to the history of Islamic medicine, see Savage-Smith E. Medicine. In: Rashed R, editor. *Encyclopaedia of the History of Arabic Science*. Vol. 3. London: Routledge, 1996: 903–62; and Ullmann M. *Islamic Medicine*. Edinburgh: Edinburgh University Press, 1978.

6   McKeown T. *The Role of Medicine*. London: Nuffield Provincial Hospitals Trust, 1976.

7   McKinlay J, McKinlay S. The questionable contribution of medical measures to the decline of mortality in the US in the twentieth century. *Milbank Memorial Fund Quarterly: Health and Society*. Summer, 1977.

8   Hume J. Rival traditions: Western medicine and yunani-tibb in the Punjab, 1849–1889. *Bulletin of the History of Medicine* 1977; 55: 24–31.

9   Gallagher N. *Medicine and Power in Tunisia*. Cambridge: Cambridge University Press, 1984.

Thinking from the USA

Chapter 9

Democratic decisions about health care: why be like NICE?*

Amy Gutmann and Dennis Thompson

'There can be no more important issue … than the workings of the National Institute for Clinical Excellence [NICE] and the implications of its workings for rationing in the health service.' With these words, Dr Evan Harris, the Liberal Democrat MP from Oxford West and Abingdon, introduced the House of Commons' first debate on the new Institute and its initial decisions.[1] NICE was created by the Government in March 1999 to provide authoritative assessments of treatments and clinical guidelines for their use.[2] The impetus for the new Institute came from the widespread recognition that the National Health Service (NHS) could not fund care for all health needs, especially the growing array of new drug treatments, and could better justify its difficult decisions if it could rely on independent advice.

Was NICE necessary? There are some purely strategic reasons why a democratic government might want to establish a body like NICE – for example, to try to distance itself from some public controversies over health care priorities. But the moral reasons for establishing NICE are more compelling, and these reasons are no less practically important than purely strategic ones. Decisions about which health care goods and services to fund for whom raise among the most morally important and difficult issues of life, quality of life, and compassion for persons. Whatever the Government's motives in establishing NICE, by appointing a respected director, members and staff, it increased its capacity for making better and fairer decisions about health care funding priorities.

Good decision-making about health care requires moral and not just strategic reasoning. Strategic reasoning shows that a decision is the best that all the

---

*   Parts of this chapter are drawn from: Just deliberation about health care. In: Clancy C, Churchill L, editors. *Ethical Dimensions of Health Policy*. Oxford: Oxford University Press, 2001; and Deliberative democracy beyond process. In: Laslett P, Fishkin J, editors. *Philosophy, Politics and Society*. Cambridge: Cambridge University Press, 2001.

decision-making parties – given their relative decision-making power – can get for themselves. It aims at striking the best bargain for the bargainers, regardless of underlying moral considerations. The obvious problem with strategic reasoning as a standard for public decision-making, especially concerning the distribution of health care, is that some people – typically not the neediest – have far greater bargaining power than others. In contrast, moral reasoning takes all similarly affected interests into account, and asks whether a decision is fair to everyone who is affected by it. Any democracy that claims to treat each citizen fairly is *ipso facto* invoking a moral justification.

When the Government established NICE, it may have been thinking strategically and hoping to avoid moral controversy, but almost as soon as NICE had been created, it came under moral attack. The debate in the Commons had hardly begun when a backbencher and physician, Dr Nick Palmer, the Labour MP from Broxtowe, tried to interrupt Harris. He wanted to challenge the idea that NICE or anyone else would be 'rationing' health care. Harris explained that he did not mean to suggest that NICE would be creating a rationing system like that used during the Second World War, where everyone 'receives a set ration of treatment that, once exhausted, cannot be used any more'. Rather, what rationing means is that 'sometimes some treatments are not available when they would benefit patients or populations, because there simply are not the resources to provide all those treatments on the NHS'. But, of course, this kind of rationing is still contentious: critics of NICE were already challenging NICE's decision, in its first review of a drug, to recommend against the NHS funding the new anti-flu drug zanamivir, marketed as Relenza by Glaxo Wellcome.[3]

The controversy surrounding the Institute and its decisions illustrates one of the most challenging set of issues in health care today: how democratic societies should make decisions about health care priorities. The debate in the House of Commons about 'the workings of NICE' and its decision against Relenza and likely future decisions is a prelude to the larger social debate in which health care professionals, politicians and citizens will be increasingly engaging in the future. The Commons debate raises questions that are typical of the kind of issues that health care decision-makers in the UK and many other democracies increasingly face. What benefits should health care plans provide and to whom? And who should have the authority to make such decisions?

In formulating policy guidance about what services the NHS should provide, NICE decision-makers act as public officials, and they therefore face many of the same challenges confronting clinicians, NHS managers or ministers. Even though the decisions made by NICE are not legally binding, they are likely to have much the same effect as Government or NHS actions. The debate in the Commons therefore is not simply about the decisions that NICE made, but about the political process in which health care decisions are made, and the standards for assessing that process. These questions go beyond NICE, because such decisions are increasingly being made or at least being influenced by many different kinds of official and unofficial bodies, such as various kinds of review boards, professional associations, ethics committees, task forces and industry councils.

Political theories of democracy suggest standards for assessing how these controversial decisions can be justifiably made. The most promising theories, we believe, defend a central role for deliberation in dealing with controversies such as those that arise in the making of health care policy. These theories of deliberative democracy offer the most promising perspective for judging health care debates because they defend a kind of politics that is explicitly designed to respond morally to moral controversies. The deliberation addresses in moral, and not just strategic, terms the public disagreements about what count as justifiable trade-offs among valued ends or between valued means and ends.

The idea of deliberative democracy

In a deliberative democracy, citizens or their accountable representatives seek to give one another mutually acceptable reasons to justify the laws and policies they adopt.[4] We call such reasons 'reciprocal' and the value they express 'reciprocity'. The reasons are not merely procedural ('because the majority favours health care') or purely substantive ('because health care is a human right'). They appeal to principles that citizens who are trying to find fair terms of co-operation can reasonably accept. Both the content of the deliberators' principles and the conditions under which they are deliberating should manifest the aim of justifying policies to the people who are bound by them. This aim may never be perfectly realised in practice, but a theory of deliberative democracy offers useful guidelines by which to judge actual decision-making as better or worse, to the extent that the reasons for the decisions are reciprocal.

Deliberation that aims at reciprocity does not necessarily guarantee a just outcome. A well-designed deliberation by NICE that considers whether to recommend NHS coverage of Relenza, the relatively inexpensive anti-influenza drug, or beta interferon, the relatively expensive drug for treating multiple sclerosis, may or may not yield a fair conclusion.[5] No decision-making process in the realm of policy-making can guarantee the right answers, since none is perfect. Deliberative processes are likely to work less well to the extent that the conditions under which they operate fail to treat people as free and equal citizens. When a political system is structured to give rich citizens far more political power than warranted by their numbers or their regard for justice, then deliberative processes will suffer. Poorer citizens will have less access to decision-makers and less decision-making power than warranted. When, in addition, the Government fails to secure an adequate level of basic opportunities – such as income and education – for all citizens, deliberative processes are likely to suffer as well.

Injustice may also result from the structure of decision-making itself – from the fact that the institutions or even the society in which the decisions are made are burdened by limits beyond their control. An example is the role of large multi-national pharmaceutical companies, which increasingly wield considerable power over governments. One of them Glaxo, the maker of Relenza, strongly urged that their drug be approved by NICE. The implicit threat, later made explicit, was that it would abandon its operations in England, which would have put many people out of work and might have led other pharmaceutical companies to boycott the UK economy. It is possible to imagine that the members of the NICE Board, after careful deliberation, backed down in face of Glaxo's threat because they reasoned that the harm that Glaxo would do to the UK economy and some of its poorest citizens would be greater than the good that would be done by standing its ground and recommending against the funding of Relenza. If the Board had approved Relenza under these conditions, we should not blame the process of deliberation itself. The problem is the context in which deliberation must occur: no matter how deliberative, NICE cannot by itself solve the problem of grossly unequal economic power. As it turned out, in this case NICE stood its ground and Glaxo backed down from its threat. Deliberation and justice coincided. But this happy ending is hardly to be expected in all cases.

When the ending is not likely to be so happy, deliberative politics has the capacity to reveal the injustice in the ending, and to suggest what justice would require. Because deliberative processes put a premium on reciprocity, they are not only more valuable in themselves than non-deliberative means but they are also more likely to come to the aid of victims of social injustice than are power-based processes of decision-making, such as interest group bargaining. In the face of unequal power, those with less are not likely to do better by bargaining than by arguing.

What kinds of reasons satisfy a standard of reciprocity? We focus here on four core characteristics of reasons that make them reciprocal. These characteristics provide standards for judging the reasons given for decisions about health care, and the institutions within which the decisions are made.[6]

Accessible reasons

First, the reasons that decision-makers give should be *accessible*. The basic rationale for the requirement is clear: if you are trying to justify imposing your will on others, your reasons should be comprehensible to them. You would expect no less from them if they were imposing their will on you. The justification, if it is to be mutual, does not even get started if those to whom it addressed cannot understand its essential content. It would not be acceptable, for example, to appeal only to the authority of revelation, whether divine or secular in nature.

Why should a similar appeal to scientific authority and expertise not also be inaccessible? Consider the justification for the decision that NICE made to recommend against the prescription of Relenza. Here is part of the reasoning from NICE's appraisal report (available on its web site).

> *The combined evidence ... indicates that the use of zanamivir (Relenza), within 48 hours from the onset of symptoms of influenza, reduces the duration of symptoms (when analysed on an intention to treat basis) from a median of 6 days to 5 days (a median reduction of 1 day, with 95% confidence intervals of 0.5 days to 1.5 days) ... From the cost of the product, alone, there is an estimated net drug cost to the NHS (based on existing estimates of the rates of primary care consultations for influenza) in a non-epidemic year of £9.9 million, and of £15 million in an epidemic year ... The impact, on primary care, of general use in the 1999/2000 influenza season is likely to be disproportionate to the benefits obtained by influenza sufferers, and is likely to distort the wider application of GP resources.[7]*

Ordinary patients – and even not so ordinary ones – may be excused if they do not fully follow this reasoning. But that does not necessarily make the justification inaccessible. The basic conclusions can be expressed in accessible terms by clarifying what the cost means (for example, by showing what other treatments might be provided for £9.9 to £15 million, and by explaining what the negative impact on primary care would be if, as predicted, many more people would make appointments to see their doctors were Relenza available). The technical knowledge and professional judgements that lie behind the conclusion not to recommend Relenza may not be unanimous, but this is true of many conclusions of experts that we reasonably accept in modern life.

Accepting the justification for such conclusions presumes a certain amount of trust – for example in some of the cost estimates – but not blind trust. The trust is not blind if two conditions hold. First, citizens have some independent basis for believing the experts are trustworthy (such as a past record of reliable judgements or a decision-making structure that contains checks and balances by experts who have reason to exercise critical scrutiny over one another). Second, the experts can describe the basis for their conclusions in way that citizens can understand. The justification, then, would be accessible in the way that reciprocity requires.

What kind of institutional arrangements would be likely to facilitate giving accessible justifications? Health care decisions are best defended in forums that include representatives of the people whose health care is in the hands of the institution. The reasons are more likely to be accessible to people if accountable representatives are present when policies are being made and defended. The NICE Board itself comprises members of the clinical professions, NHS managers and research bodies, and some representatives from patients and user groups. But the vast majority of members are health care professionals. The Partner's Council of NICE includes all the key stakeholder groups and many more representatives of patients (as well as health professionals, NHS officials, and members of the health care industry). This Council may therefore go further toward filling the deliberative requirement that the process should involve representatives of the people whose health care is in the hands of the NHS.

It is too early to say how well the Partner's Council will work in tandem with the NICE Board (which has greater day-to-day decision-making power). The key factor that would affect whether the arrangement satisfies the conditions of accessibility depends on the membership of the Partner's Council and on the co-operation of this body and the NICE Board. The representatives on the Partner's Council should include people who have some typical experiences in receiving health care services through the NHS or have very close contact with people who do. They should routinely be encouraged to ask critical questions of NICE and to challenge answers until the reasoning satisfies them.

In light of the generally greater power of health care institutions than their patient base, institutions like NICE should be required to give reasons for their policies to a body that can act as a patient tribune, jury or ombudsman. Among other responsibilities, the patient tribune would make sure that the explanations the experts give on behalf of the institution are comprehensible to the patient representatives. Representatives should have access to records of the past decisions and qualifications of the major decision-makers. Detailed technical material supporting the justification of decisions, such as whether to recommend prescribing Relenza, should also be available for evaluation by independent experts. Individual patients or their representatives should be able to consult independent experts as a check on the reliability of the organisation's experts, whose judgement about what counts as a reasonable and affordable health care risk may be unintentionally skewed in some way. This bias may discovered only by considering technical details that are beyond what patients or their representatives are able to analyse on their own.

Moral reasons

Reciprocity demands more than accessible reasons. Self-interested reasons – reasons that serve the interests of a particular interest group, such as a single employer or a single drug company – are conspicuously accessible. In contrast to self-interested reasons, reciprocity presumes a moral point of view. What counts as a moral reason? The basic criterion of a moral reason – sometimes called 'generality' – is one that deliberative democracy shares with many other moral and political theories. The criterion of generality is so widely accepted that it is often identified with the moral point of view.[8] Moral arguments apply to everyone who is similarly situated in the morally relevant respects. Patients who ask to have access to the use of beta interferon for the symptomatic treatment of their multiple sclerosis – a treatment that costs about £10,000 per year – do not, if acting morally, assert that only some patients with their symptoms should have such access (or that only NHS doctors in some regions who treat such patients should be financially able to prescribe beta interferon). Rather, they assert that all patients with similar symptoms and similarly receptivity to the treatment should have access to it (and all doctors who treat such patients should be financially able to prescribe it).

In the debate in the House of Commons, James Gray, the MP from North Wiltshire, implicitly appealed to generality – the moral idea that like cases should be treated alike – when he complained that even though some citizens in other parts of the country could get beta interferon from the NHS, his constituents could not. This, he noted, is 'a terrible tragedy for constituents such as mine, who could be prescribed beta interferon if they lived in Bath or Oxford, but not in Wiltshire'.[9] However, generality does not always lead to a positive conclusion: when NICE decided against Relenza, it did so for reasons that are general in this moral sense. NICE stressed that the benefit to *all* patients of influenza 'is modest and on the present evidence is restricted to reducing the symptoms of influenza by one day [while] the costs of achieving this benefit … will be significant'.

Generality always raises a substantive question: what are the morally relevant respects in which people are similarly situated? The debate in the Commons shows clearly that generality is not a purely formal standard. One possible moral response to arguments against prescribing Relenza for all people who have influenza is to recommend prescription for patients who are particularly at risk of complications arising from influenza. NICE addressed this possibility in its report when it asked: [10]

> … *whether zanamivir (Relenza) should be prescribed to 'high risk' patients. In the absence of clear evidence of benefit in reducing the serious secondary complications of influenza, in such individuals, the Institute did not regard it as appropriate for zanamivir (Relenza) to be offered to 'high risk' patients.*

NICE went on to call for more research on the effects of Relenza on high-risk patients. This recommendation too was, or could be, justified in general terms. A morally relevant characteristic – being at high risk of complications from influenza – was applied generally. There may also be morally justified general reasons for not spending public money on additional research on Relenza, rather than on some other, more promising drug. A reason that qualifies as moral by deliberative standards may be opposed by another moral reason. Moral reasoning therefore leaves room for reasonable disagreement because moral reasons may be multiple and may support opposing policy conclusions.

Institutions like NICE should be designed to encourage more moral rather than more self-interested reasoning and action. Forums for deliberation that include representatives of less advantaged citizens encourage decision-makers to take a broader perspective on the matters that come before them. Deliberation will not turn self-centred individualists suddenly into public-spirited citizens. The NICE Board – including as it does clinical professionals, academics, NHS managers, patients, and user groups – is designed so that its members should not think of themselves as representatives of special interest groups. The Partners' Council spans a broader range of constituencies: its members include representatives of patients, care givers, pharmaceutical companies, and other health care industries. Although the Partners' Council, by its criteria of participation, invites members to think as representatives, it too depends on its members' thinking in moral rather than self-interested, or group-interested, terms.

How can deliberative forums provide incentives for moral reasoning? The forums are likely to work best when they are designed to reproduce as little as possible the processes of power politics and interest group bargaining. Members of the NICE Board, as its charter suggests, should not think of themselves as merely group-interested delegates, even if they inevitably and quite properly bring different perspectives to the meetings. The same proviso applies to the Partners' Council. In both cases, the membership should not be chosen in a way that suggests that each represents the interests of a single constituent group, whose interests the member is therefore bound to articulate and promote. A forum that is so organised is likely to reproduce the results of interest group bargaining, and discourage the processes of moral reasoning.

From this perspective, the structure of the NICE Board and the Partners' Council – because they bring together people from different backgrounds – is far better than the committee structures of most Health Maintenance Organisations (HMOs) in the USA, where, typically, separate medical committees, benefit committees and consumer affairs committees each concentrate on a different aspect of the policy and are therefore encouraged to engage in a process of decision-making that more closely resembles interest group bargaining.[11] When committees are structured as interest groups, they are more likely to advocate a position that reflects their own special perspective or particular interest. They arrive at policy conclusions without much exposure to the perspectives or interests represented by the other committees.

The Partners' Council has a wide-ranging membership, but the crucial factor is how often the Council will meet and how actively it will therefore deliberate about the recommendations by the NICE Board before they are implemented. Initial statements suggested that the Council would merely review the NICE's progress and issue annual reports. There were no indications that the Council would be a forceful body. By contrast, the NICE Board – which is the primary decision-making body – meets frequently, has the opportunity to engage in a great deal of deliberation, but also has very few members who are not health care professionals. It would be better, from the perspective of moral reasoning, if the forum in which final decisions are made included more voices that reflect as many relevant perspectives as feasible.

For what reasons, and to what extent, if at all, should NICE take into account the limited resources available at any given time to the NHS? If NICE is to maintain public support and confidence, its Board members must be able to offer publicly defensible answers to these questions, and such answers must rely on moral reasoning. This is not to say that moral reasoning offers one and only one answer, but it is to deny that the strategic reasoning offers a wholly adequate answer.

Respectful reasons

Another virtue of the deliberative conception of decision-making is that it recognises that much moral disagreement will persist even among intelligent and good-willed people. Some of the moral disagreement that persists about public policy is reasonable: it is moral and there is no morally definitive perspective that for public purposes settles the disagreement. Health care policy poses some of the most intractable of these issues. Should individuals be held responsible for health problems that are partly the product of their own choices? Should children who cannot give informed consent ever be subjects of experimental medical research? Should health care treatments be publicly funded when they marginally improve quality of life but are not judged to be cost-effective by most health care experts and yet will be affordable (and therefore purchased) by more affluent citizens? The answers to these questions depend significantly on moral considerations, and even while agreeing on the facts, different people are likely to answer them differently. The problem, from a public perspective, is that our answers more often than not conflict, and some of the conflicts will be moral and reasonable.

In face of disagreement of this kind, the deliberative conception specifies a third criterion of reasoning, also intended to encourage reciprocity: the reasons that decision-makers give should be *mutually respectful* of those who are similarly striving for mutual respect. Mutual respect demands more than toleration or a benign attitude of indifference towards others. It requires a favourable attitude toward, and constructive interaction with, people with whom one reasonably disagrees when those persons are similarly willing and able to adopt such an attitude. In respecting one another as moral agents, participants in a deliberative process recognise the difference between morally respectable differences of opinion and merely tolerable ones. Differences that represent morally respectable conflicts are what we call 'deliberative disagreements': conflicts in which citizens seek a resolution that is mutually justifiable but differ about moral principles or their practical implications.

Many disputes about how much emphasis to place on individual responsibility for certain health care problems, or how much value to place on very marginal improvements in quality of life, and how much consumers therefore should be required to bear some of the costs of their health care, are examples of deliberative disagreements. Conflicting sides can justify their views as reasonable within a reciprocal perspective. In contrast, consider a dispute in which some people criticise and others defend denying health care to individuals on grounds of race or religion. This would be an example of a non-deliberative disagreement, because one side can be rejected as unreasonable within a reciprocal perspective.[12] This side rejects the very premise of reciprocity – the idea that mutually binding laws and policies should be mutually justified to the people who will be bound by them. Discrimination on grounds of race or religion cannot be justified to those who are disadvantaged by these policies.

In a deliberative process characterised by mutual respect, participants recognise the moral merit in their opponents' claims (insofar as they have merit). Such a process can help clarify what is at stake in a moral disagreement by encouraging deliberators to sort out self-interested claims from public-spirited ones and to recognise those public-spirited claims that should have greater weight. Through a deliberative process, participants in a health care forum can isolate those conflicts that embody genuinely incompatible values on both sides. Conflicts that do not involve such deep disagreement can then be easily addressed and may turn out to be more resolvable than they appeared at first sight. Some may be the result of misunderstanding or lack of information, and some may be appropriately settled by bargaining, negotiation and compromise. In this way, deliberation helps put moral principle and moral compromise, bargaining and compromise in their place.

In the face of deliberative disagreements, deliberative democracy recommends what we call an 'economy of moral disagreement'. In justifying policies on moral grounds, citizens should seek the rationale that minimises rejection of the position they oppose. By economising on their disagreements in this way, citizens manifest mutual respect as they continue to disagree about morally important issues on which they need to reach collective decisions.

In the spirit of economising on moral disagreement, proponents of NICE could acknowledge that the Institute is aiding the NHS in making hard choices among health care treatments under a limited budget. If this is all that 'rationing' means, then it was not publicly productive to denounce or even criticise one's opponents for using the term 'rationing'. In the same spirit, the critics of NICE's decisions should, in turn, be able to agree not to use the term 'rationing' as a scare word. Everyone today should be able to agree that it is fiscally impossible for any society to fund every single health care treatment that has some marginal benefit to some people, regardless of its cost or cost-effectiveness.

The Commons debate over the role of NICE has little to gain but obfuscation if it focuses on whether 'NICE is about rational thinking and not rationing of treatment'. NICE is about both. NICE's reasoning about Relenza is rational thinking about public funding of a health care treatment. NICE's reasoning about Relenza is also about setting publicly defensible limits on which health care treatments will be publicly funded. There is a serious debate to be had on what treatments should be publicly funded and why. Whatever public officials of different parties call the practice of limiting public funding, they should be able to agree that health care resources are limited and should be used in a publicly effective and publicly defensible way.

Economising on moral disagreement means that participants in the debate should try to set aside contentious issues on which further discussion is not likely to clarify the disagreement, and concentrate on issues on which discussion is likely to reveal substantive moral differences, even if it will not produce agreement. In the Commons debate, Dr Harris raised again the issue of rationing. To deny that NICE would be supporting the NHS's rationing of drugs would be like saying, 'the earth is flat'. Although some of his opponents took him up on the call for another debate on 'rationing', the more productive (and deliberative) response was to focus on the more substantive point he sought to make. What he really objected to was not rationing *per se*, but what he regarded as unfairness. He believed that the decision not to cover Relenza discriminated against poor people: 'When we talk about rationing of NHS treatments, we aren't saying no one in the UK has them. What we are saying is that they aren't available to poor people. The rich and those who can afford it can get these treatments privately.' The money saved for all patients would be at the expense of the poor because more affluent citizens could obtain Relenza by private means or by moving to a part of the country where Relenza is available through postcode prescribing (which reflects the decisions of some health authorities to provide health care above and beyond that offered in other regions). The decision by NICE to recommend against prescribing Relenza would, therefore, at least appear to be sacrificing the welfare of some poorer citizens in order to save taxpayer money.

Suppose that Parliament had never conducted a debate about NICE. Or suppose that NICE had recommended against prescribing Relenza with no public comment. In either case, advocates of funding Relenza could reasonably have thought that NICE was putting cost savings for UK taxpayers above concern for the health of poor citizens. Regardless of whether a decision not to fund Relenza was right, a defence of NICE's decision on the narrow technical merits without the wider moral debate would have failed to appreciate the value of respectful reasons.

Whatever the merits of Dr Harris' criticism, all parties to the dispute over Relenza should be able to agree that he has raised a serious moral question. Even if, under current conditions, the NHS cannot do anything about this differential access to drugs such as Relenza, defenders of the decision (and other similarly hard choices) should be prepared to acknowledge the moral costs inherent in a situation in which rich people can buy any health care treatment on the market whereas poor people are completely dependent on the NHS for funding those treatments that may be cost-effective for society as a whole.

Although economising on moral disagreement may sometimes reduce moral conflict, it does not eliminate it. Indeed, in the process of clarifying and identifying moral differences, it may intensify it. Some critics of mutual respect therefore may object that deliberative practices raise the moral stakes. Suppose that NHS doctors had rejected the recommendation of NICE about Relenza. The political conflict might then have become greater than it would have been without any deliberation. Had this happened, the NHS might have rued the day that NICE was created. Critics of deliberation are correct in suggesting that in some contexts the effort to economise on moral disagreement may turn what would otherwise be a simple bargaining situation into a conflict of moral principle, and thereby encourage no-holds-barred opposition and political intransigence.

But many issues, especially in the realm of health care, are already morally sensitive. And if the controversy is temporarily suppressed through some political compromise, it is likely to erupt again. Deliberation does not usually create moral controversy, and though it may sometimes intensify the conflict, it can also in the process clarify what is at stake, so that opponents can separate their resolvable from their irresolvable differences. More importantly, avoiding moral arguments may have the effect of obscuring injustice. When a dispute raises serious moral issues – the avoidable deaths of less-affluent patients or the exclusion of certain groups such as immigrants, for example – then it is not likely to be resolved more satisfactorily by avoiding arguments that are both moral and mutually respectful. Most disputes in health care raise serious moral issues and therefore put a social premium on parties' mutually seeking an economy of moral disagreement.

Revisable reasons

A fourth fundamental feature of reciprocal reasoning is that its conclusions are *morally revisable* over time. Decision-makers who render complex and controversial decisions, about which there are reasonable disagreements, should seek to maintain opportunities for others to challenge and to revise their decision in the future, in light of new scientific information, fresh understandings of the moral values at stake, and other changes in the context within which the decision is made. When the NICE Board ruled against Relenza, it implicitly recognised this criterion of revisability. At the same time that it recommended that Relenza should not be funded in the forthcoming influenza season, it also recommended that additional trials be conducted and further data be obtained.

Particular attention, the Board said, should be paid to two critical issues. First, we need to know whether Relenza has positive effects on reducing serious secondary complications of influenza in 'high-risk' patients. Second, we must seek better estimates of the costs of prescribing Relenza – the direct costs as well as the indirect costs from the increased use of primary care physicians. Recall that one reason that NICE recommended against Relenza was the concern that primary care physicians would be overwhelmed with appointments by influenza patients when they could be seeing patients with more medically serious and treatable ailments. If it turns out that primary care physicians end up seeing nearly as many influenza patients as expected with Relenza, or if additional clinical trials reveal greater benefits than now expected from its prescription, then by calling for more studies NICE, in effect, declares that it stands ready to reconsider its decision for future influenza seasons.

The moral basis of the criterion of revisability is the value of reciprocity. Decision-makers owe moral justifications for the policies that they seek to impose on other people. If they take seriously their opponents' moral reasons, they must acknowledge the possibility that, at least for a certain range of views, their opponents may be shown to be correct in the future. This possibility has implications not only for the way citizens should treat their opponents but also for the way they should regard their own views. If they act on the idea of revisability, they will continually test their own views, seeking forums in which the views can be challenged, and keeping open the possibility of their revision or even rejection. Deliberative forums that deal with moral disagreements put a premium on presenting justifications in a way that can stand the test of new moral insights, empirical evidence, and alternative interpretations of insights and evidence.

The purpose of revisability is not only to respect the moral status of the participants in the process but also to improve the quality of the decisions that they make. Revisability offers important protection against the mistakes that citizens, politicians and health care professionals all inevitably make. Ideally, all participants in the decision-making process recognise that their reasons and conclusions should be revisable. But even when some or all of the participants do not share this recognition, a well-constituted deliberative forum can foster revisability.

In an institution designed to encourage deliberation, participants have an incentive to learn from each other, to rectify their individual and collective misapprehensions, and to develop new views and policies that can more successfully withstand each other's critical scrutiny. When citizens bargain and negotiate, they may learn how better to get what they wanted to begin with. But when they deliberate, they may instead learn how to want something better, that they did *not* want to begin with.

For health care institutions, the most important implication of the revisability criterion is that decision-making bodies should be designed so that their conclusions are regarded as provisional. Medical findings that are relevant to health care decisions change rapidly and sometimes dramatically over time. The economic conditions of society that are relevant to the resources available to health care institutions also vary. What counts as adequate health care depends on objective as well as subjective social conditions. And changes in one institution – such as government policy made in Parliament – are relevant to other institutions – such as the decisions made by NICE and the NHS.

At any given time, deliberative forums, of course, must reach conclusions, but the conclusions should always be open to challenge in a subsequent round of deliberation. Deliberation continues through stages, as various health care officials present their proposals, consumers respond, officials revise, consumers react, and the stages recur. This is what we call the 'reiteration of deliberation', which also recommends deliberative democracy and makes it more suitable to decision-making under conditions of shifting uncertainties.

The potential strengths (and shortcomings) of this kind of deliberation can be seen in NICE's decision-making process for setting health care priorities, as brought out in the Commons debate. Several MPs objected that NICE should not be using affordability as a criterion for deciding whether to recommend that the NHS prescribes a treatment. Mrs Caroline Spelman, the Conservative member from Meriden, argued that for NICE to take account of affordability, is 'to shield the Government from the very difficult decisions that have to be taken'. As an appointed body, NICE is less directly accountable to UK citizens. Dr Harris expressed a similar concern when he argued that affordability was a matter for the Government [not NICE] to decide. Should NICE recommend beta interferon, which costs about £10,000 per patient per year, and has been judged 'marginally effective'? (It treats incurable multiple sclerosis 'by reducing the exacerbation rate in patients who have relapsing-remitting disease without important disability'.[13]) Should NICE recommend the new taxane drugs for chemotherapy that do not cure but, as Dr Harris put it, 'can add years to life at a cost of about £10,000 per year'?

If NICE recommends against prescribing expensive new drugs that can provide some health care benefits to patients, will they thereby be shielding the Government from pressure to increase the total NHS budget? If NICE recommends in favour of the NHS prescribing all or some of these drugs, will they thereby be forcing the NHS not to fund some other existing and highly valuable treatments (or pressuring the Government to increase funding for the NHS)? Harris is surely correct in insisting that the choice has to be recognised. Those who voiced criticism of NICE in the debate are correct in claiming that these are not issues 'on which the Government should hide behind NICE'. Non-elective institutions such as NICE should not be used to shield the Government from making hard choices or from justifying those choices to UK citizens, the people who will be bound by them.

But such concerns should not be overstated. NICE's decisions are not likely to be taken as the final word, and are just as likely to begin the debate as to conclude it on any particular issue. To be sure, NICE's decisions at any given time have important consequences, first and foremost for patients who depend exclusively on the NHS for their health care. But among the other consequences of NICE's decisions at any given time may be an increase in pressure on the Government to face up to the hard choices that it needs to make when expensive new treatments come on the global market. When deliberative forums persist over time, and provide continuing opportunities for challenge, they encourage the reiteration of deliberation. The Commons debate that we have been following here is itself a stage in this reiterative process. Such debates lessen the danger that the Government will avoid making hard choices, or will try to make them without the benefit of full public discussion.

NICE should be as clear as possible about whether it is assuming that the NHS budget is a constant, or whether it is calling for a change in its budget in order to fund a certain treatment. If NICE's assumptions are clear, then its recommendation – for or against prescribing a particular treatment – will not shield the Government from the responsibility of either accepting or rejecting the constraints under which NICE's recommendation is being made. When NICE makes decisions that are revisable – and revisable not only by NICE but also by the Government when it decides to spend more or less money on health care – then the basis of the hard choices that are made about health care becomes more explicit, and the decision-makers more accountable.

Conclusion

Hard choices in health care that were once made largely behind closed doors, with very little public appreciation of the need to set priorities and accept limits, are now more often being made in open forums, where decision-makers have to justify their actions and respond to objections raised by citizens and their representatives. Such deliberations have the potential to help citizens, legislators and health care professionals come to a better understanding of their own values – those they share and those they do not. Deliberating about hard choices in health care, over time and in multiple public forums, can help citizens and their elected and appointed representatives undertake, in a more reciprocal spirit, what is likely to be a long and difficult process of setting and revising priorities that will affect the quality of health care both now and in the future.

If the values of deliberative democracy are to be more fully realised in the practices of health care forums, the justifications that the decision-makers give should be more accessible, moral, respectful and revisable. To the extent that the institutions for making these decisions are in these ways deliberation-friendly, the decisions that they produce will be more reciprocal, and the health care policies they represent will be more morally legitimate even if they are not always politically popular. By making the process in which citizens decide the future of their health care more deliberative, they stand a better chance of resolving some of their moral disagreements, and living on reciprocal terms with those that inevitably persist.

References

1   House of Commons Debates. *Hansard*; 10 November 1999: col 1066–88.
2   See statements by NICE's newly appointed director, Michael Rawlins: Horton R. NICE: A step forward in the quality of NHS care. *Lancet* 1999; 353: 1028–9; and Yamey G. Chairman of NICE admits that its judgments are hard to defend. *BMJ* 1999; 319: 1222.
3   See: NICE appraisal of Zanamivir (Relenza). Posted at www.nice.org.uk. For some of the reaction, see Moore S D. UK rebuffs Glaxo on new flu drug. *Wall Street Journal* 1999; October 11: A19.
4   This conception of democracy including the value of that we present here is developed more systematically in Gutmann A, Thompson D. *Democracy and Disagreement*. Cambridge: Belknap Press of Harvard University Press, 1996.
5   On interferons, see Walley T, Barton S. A purchaser perspective of managing new drugs; inteferon beta as a case study. *BMJ* 1995; 311: 796–99; and Rous E *et al*. A purchaser experience of managing new expensive drugs: interferon beta. *BMJ* 1996; 313: 1195–6.
6   These criteria should be regarded as necessary conditions (which can be satisfied to varying degrees). For other criteria that specify the conditions of deliberation, such as publicity and accountability, see Gutmann A and Thompson D, above, pp. 95–164.
7   See the Institute's web site: www.nice.org.uk
8   See Baier K. *The Moral Point of View*. Ithaca: Cornell University Press, 1958: 187–213; and Rawls J. *A Theory of Justice*. Cambridge: Harvard, 1971: 130–6.
9   This criticism implicitly raises questions about the relative degree of autonomy that local health authorities should have in setting priorities. See Lenaghan J. The rationing debate: central government should have a greater role in rationing decisions. *BMJ* 1997; 314: 967–71.
10   NICE Appraisal of Zanamivir (Relenza). Posted at www.nice.org.uk
11   See for example Karen G, Gervais *et al*., editors. *Ethical Challenges in Managed Care*. Washington, DC: Georgetown University Press, 1999: chapter 1.
12   See Gutmann and Thompson, above pp. 2–3, 73–9.
13   Rous *et al*. above, pp. 1195–6.

Chapter 10

The trade-off between equity and choice: ensuring fair procedures

Dan W Brock

In the design of any health care system, different values that we seek to achieve and respect will inevitably come into conflict. One central value in health care system design is equity, which I shall understand here as the fair distribution of the benefits and burdens of the health care system. Equity concerns the comparative treatment of different individuals or groups within the health care system and whether the differences in their treatment are morally justified or just. A second fundamental value in health care system design is individual choice. This chapter explores briefly the nature of these two values and their ethical importance, and then takes up some different contexts in which they come into conflict in a health care system. We will see that different individual choices have different ethical importance and raise more or less serious conflicts with equity, as well as with other values. Since both theories of justice and reasonable people often disagree about how to resolve these conflicts and make the necessary trade-offs, I shall then argue that a fair and democratic resolution of them must rely principally on fair procedures that reflect the diverse views of individuals about the trade-offs and give due regard to individuals' concerns and interests.

I would emphasise at the outset that the conflict between equity and choice and the necessary trade-offs that it requires is intrinsic to any health care system, and not special to the National Health Service (NHS). In the systematic health care reform proposal of the Clinton administration in the USA in the early 1990s, in whose development I took part, we also sought to identify the underlying ethical principles and values that guided that health care reform and the inevitable trade-offs between them in the design of the system.[1] There, too, we identified the conflict between maximising individual choice, on the one hand, and equity and efficiency in the health care system, on the other. Because of the differences in the structure of that proposed health care system and the NHS, the specific detailed institutional conflicts and trade-offs between equity and choice will differ, but the fundamental ethical and value conflicts are largely the same.

In the UK, the trade-off between equity and choice has often been seen over the last two decades in the broader political context of debates concerning privatisation of various aspects of the health care system and efforts to introduce market reforms into the NHS. Many people associate respecting individual choice, both in the health care system and elsewhere, with promoting the use of private markets to provide and distribute goods and services. The fundamental idea is that markets maximise the ability of individuals to act on their own individual preferences and desires, and so markets are thought maximally to reflect and respect differences in the preferences and choices of individuals in the use of their resources, and more generally in the pursuit of their inevitably differing values and conceptions of a good life. While there is an important element of truth in this association of choice and market reforms, I shall argue that it is oversimplified and mistaken in a number of important respects. But for now it is sufficient to point out that probably the most important change in health care systems in many countries, including the UK, over the last several decades in increasing individual choice was not a change fundamentally associated with the introduction of private markets. Instead, it was the broad change in the normative understanding of the physician–patient relationship, and in particular of the roles of physicians and patients in medical treatment decision-making.

From a largely authoritarian or paternalist understanding of the physician–patient relationship that was dominant in most countries several decades ago, we have moved to a model of shared decision-making between physicians and patients. In the earlier paternalist model, the physician was seen as the proper decision-maker about treatment, with the patient's role largely one of complying with the physician's orders. In the newer model of shared decision-making, physicians, of course, still have an important role in informing patients about their diagnosis, prognosis, and treatment alternatives with their respective risks and benefits, but now patients have a new more active role in making informed choices from among those alternatives according to their own values.[2] It is now widely recognised in many countries that competent patients have the right to refuse any treatment and to select from among available alternative treatments. This change in the norm for treatment decision-making, while still incomplete in practice in all countries, has nevertheless transformed physician–patient relationships and has gone a long way to increase respecting patients' choice of their health care.

The point to be emphasised here is that this change is not principally the result of greater use of private markets within health care, but rather has been grounded in an increasing appreciation of the importance of individual self-determination or autonomy in medical decision-making and in the design of health care systems. It reflects the increased importance given to this value, not the greater role of private markets or increased privatisation within health care systems. The importance of individual choice in health care system design should be recognised across the liberal–conservative political spectrum, and it remains an open question whether and to what extent specific privatisation and market reforms will better respect individual self-determination or autonomy in the health care system.

Equity

I have said that equity concerns the fair or just distribution of the benefits and burdens of the health care system, but have said nothing about what constitutes a fair or just distribution. Giving a detailed specification of a particular account of equity would be extremely complex and controversial, and will not be attempted here. Doing so would require developing standards for prioritising different claims on inevitably scarce health care resources. What weight should be given to such considerations as severity and urgency of need, degree of expected benefit, cost, and so forth? These and other considerations all bear on the equitable distribution of health benefits and costs for individuals from different allocations of resources, and people reasonably disagree about what weight to give them in health care resource prioritisation. However, there is widespread agreement that need should be at least a central distribution criterion, and that simply distributing health care according to ability to pay is not equitable, most importantly because it leaves the urgent health care needs of many persons unmet. If maximising individual choice is associated with maximising the use of markets for the distribution of health care, which I have argued above is mistaken, then the conflict between equity and individual choice would be stark indeed, since fully respecting individual choice through private markets would distribute health care according to ability to pay and without reference to health care needs.

Choice

Individual choice, or more generally individual self-determination or autonomy, are values we seek to respect in many areas of life. People's interest in self-determination is the interest of ordinary persons in making important decisions about their lives for themselves and according to their own values or conception of a good life, not according to what someone else believes would be best for them. It is through the exercise of individual self-determination and having it respected by others that we take control of and responsibility for our own lives. It is this capacity for individual agency and, in turn, responsibility, that is an important source of human dignity. All choices are not equally important to people, however, and it is worth underlining why choice in the health care system is often of special importance. Perhaps the most significant feature affecting the importance of individuals' different choices is the extent of the impact of those choices on their lives. Serious disease and illness typically affect our lives in deeply personal and far reaching ways, often greatly changing the nature and direction of our lives, or even resulting in the end of our lives. The profound effects of many health care choices, especially when we are seriously ill, make it especially important to most individuals to be able to control their health care. Thus, properly respecting individual choice can be especially important in the context of providing health care, but we need also to differentiate some distinct elements of choice within a health care system. I believe there are three main elements of individual choice that should be distinguished here: choice of the health care plan or system in which one receives treatment; choice of individual physicians and other health care professionals who provide treatment; and choice of the treatment that will be provided. We will look at each of these elements of choice in turn.

Choice of health plans

The choice of health plans from which to receive one's care may not seem to be an issue in the UK, with a national health plan such as the NHS. By contrast, in a country such as the USA, in which there are many different health plans and delivery systems that differ widely in organisation, scope, and quality of services, the choice of a health plan is sometimes the most important choice individuals make in determining the nature and quality of care that they ultimately receive. Increased use of competition within the NHS and such practices as provider groups taking on financial risks, may create significant differences in the nature and quality of care received from different groups or sectors within the NHS. The greater the differences in the nature and quality of care across different parts of the NHS, the more important it can be to provide patients with significant choice of where within the NHS they receive care. However, since access and quality differences within the NHS will often be associated with geographical location, providing significant choice may be difficult or impossible when individuals are tied to particular geographical areas. This speaks strongly for limiting, on grounds of equity, differences in the nature and quality of care available within the NHS itself.

There is one choice concerning the health plan or system from which one will receive care that has become increasingly important in the UK in the last couple of decades – the choice of whether to obtain care within the NHS or to exit the NHS and seek privately purchased care or private health insurance. Without at least a perception of significant differences in the nature, quality, or timeliness of care available in the public and private sectors, people would have little incentive to exit the public sector, where care can be obtained without significant out-of-pocket costs, to the private sector in which it cannot. If the private sector does have advantages in the nature, quality or timeliness of care that would warrant individuals exiting the public sector in favour of the private sector, how serious is the inequity that is created by these differences in the care available based on the ability to pay rather than need? Clearly, other things being equal, the greater the differences in the nature, quality and timeliness of services, the greater the potential inequity. More specifically, the inequity will be more serious the more that the care available in the NHS fails to meet a reasonable standard of adequacy.

So long as the large majority of citizens continue to receive care within the NHS that they judge to be generally adequate, the presence of a smaller private system into which a minority of the better-off members of the population exit will constitute what I would characterise as an 'inequality at the top'. That is, a small portion of the population will be getting additional or better-quality services, but not sufficiently more or better quality as to seriously impact their overall well-being in comparison with the services available to all. The fact that the great majority of the population receives care through the NHS creates strong political pressure to keep that care at a level that the population judges to be adequate. This is to be contrasted with the 'inequality at the bottom' which exists in a country such as the USA, where about 15 per cent of the population lacks health insurance and so does not have a regular and reliable source of access to even basic health care services. Inequality at the bottom is more inequitable because it is the worse-off members of the population, at least with regard to access to health care services, who are without even basic, as opposed to marginally beneficial, care and services, and because being a worse-off minority rather than majority, they will be less able politically to assure that they receive even minimally adequate services. In comparison with countries in which there is no effective private sector alternative to a national health system, the presence of the exit option to the private sector in the UK, while it does produce some inequity in health care, can have a desirable competitive effect in providing incentives to improve services within the NHS. But this effect is only likely to be positive to the extent that funding for the NHS is adequate to enable it to provide a reasonable level of services.

Choice of health care providers

The second important area of choice for individuals in the design of their health care system is the choice of their providers, in particular the choice of physicians. The fear of loss of this choice was a strong source of opposition to the Clinton health care reform proposal, though the subsequent growth of managed care in the USA has eroded this choice substantially as well. Why should the choice of their health care provider be important to patients? One obvious answer is that providers often differ in the quality of services that they deliver to patients. But beyond this, and at least as important to many patients, is the fact that the physician–patient relationship can often be quite personal, intimate and long term, in which trust is important to its effective functioning, and in which it is important for patients to feel unconstrained in providing full information relevant to their care to their physicians. For a variety of reasons, a relationship of mutual understanding, respect and comfort can contribute to good health outcomes for patients. This can be especially true in the case of primary care physicians, where the relationship will often build up over time and where personal qualities in the relationship are often important to its success. Relationships with specialist physicians involved in the care of chronic illness can also have this long-term nature, where trust, respect and comfort in the relationship can again significantly enhance health outcomes. Choice of specialist physicians can be particularly important to patients when they perceive that there are serious health issues at stake, and so differences in the nature and quality of their physicians and the care they provide may be extremely important to the patient's well-being.

Reasonable choice of physicians can generally be achieved without substantial sacrifice of other values that are important in the health care system. Often this will simply require attention to the importance of ensuring some choice of individual physicians and other health professionals, and then instituting arrangements which make such choices reasonably available to patients. But there can be conflicts and trade-offs with other values. For example, in order to increase the choice of physicians, especially specialist physicians, it may be necessary to concentrate larger numbers of physicians in a single facility. This can have the consequence of creating large differences in travel times, costs and burdens for patients who live at different distances from the facility. Since equity concerns not just the distribution of health benefits, but also the burdens of obtaining those benefits, this can amount to a serious inequity which can in turn impact on quality of care. This example displays, in addition, that the trade-offs required to ensure reasonable choice of physicians can go beyond simply the conflict with equity. Data show that, especially for complex surgical procedures, quality of outcomes, both in morbidity and mortality, improve substantially with the frequency with which specialists undertake the procedures. Thus, the decision about the degree to which facilities and specialists are concentrated or dispersed can affect not just choice and equity, but also health outcomes. As with other concrete trade-offs, reasonable people can disagree about how to balance different values regarding the degree to which facilities and physicians should be concentrated or dispersed geographically. Providing greater choice of physicians can also conflict with equity to the extent that the middle and upper classes are able to 'work' the system more successfully in their favour, because they are either more articulate or better informed about how the system functions.

Choice of treatments

I believe the most important area of choice for patients is the choice of treatments that they will receive within the health care system. The paramount importance of this choice is perhaps best seen in contemplating what would be involved in denying it. We could imagine physicians making judgements about what treatment would be best for a given patient and then authorised to force that treatment on even a competent patient who refuses it. This would violate the firmly grounded moral and legal right of competent patients to give or withhold informed consent to their own treatment. The importance of informed consent is both to respect patients' self-determination or autonomy, but also to help determine which treatment would be best for a particular patient. As medical science and its clinical application have advanced in recent decades, increasing numbers of patients face numerous alternative treatments, all of which are within the bounds of medical acceptability and none of which will be best for all patients. One important reason for shared decision-making between physicians and patients is the necessity to involve the patient in the determination of what treatment will be best for him or her, a decision that can often only be reached with input from the patient about his or her particular concerns and values that bear on the choice.

Moreover, in clinical decision-making, patients may sometime reasonably choose not to attempt to maximise their health at the cost of their other aims and concerns; this can lead to choices that conflict with efficiency and cost-effectiveness in the health care system, but that nevertheless reasonably accord with patients' overall well-being and plans of life. This implies that treatment guidelines or algorithms for particular medical conditions, which have the important benefit of helping make clinical medicine more evidence based and in turn health maximising, need at the same time to be flexible enough to respect reasonable differences in the choices that individual patients make about their treatment. There is also an important tension between respecting individual choice and the efficient production of health improvements when patients choose various forms of 'alternative medicine' for which there is little or no evidence supporting its efficacy. The health care system can appropriately limit choice by imposing reasonable standards of established efficacy for what will be provided in the health care system from public funds, but needs to do so while being sensitive to the trade-off with individual choice and the preferences of patients.

The most important tension between equity and choice arises from the limits on access to beneficial treatments any plausible account of equity requires; budget limits necessitated by the importance of meeting other non-health needs and desires from either governmental or individual resources require health care rationing. Health is one among other goods, not the only good in life, and so resources need to be available for other purposes as well as health care. Unconstrained choices of treatments by patients without any resource limits would lead to the use of any health care with any positive expected benefit, no matter how small the benefit and how high the costs; this would be irrational and would exceed any plausible account of reasonable or equitable resource limits. It would also make it impossible to implement any judgement about an equitable distribution of resources between patients. Properly respecting individual choice by patients does not require meeting unlimited demands on public resources within the NHS. But it does put ethical constraints on how these limits on available treatment are determined and implemented. Detailed substantive standards for rationing decisions and the prioritisation of limited health care resources are inherently controversial – the controversies reflect deeper controversies about the relative importance of different health care services and benefits, and about distributive justice more generally.

Rationing and fair procedures

We lack sufficient consensus, either among the general public or within theories of distributive justice, on the determinate standards necessary for detailed rationing decisions and prioritisation of health care resources, and so must rely in significant part on fair procedures which ensure that people's different and conflicting interests and perspectives are properly reflected in making these decisions.[3] I want to suggest here four principles that I believe are central to such procedures being fair. Collectively, these principles are designed to balance, in an appropriate way, the importance of individual choice about treatment with the necessity for just limits on health care resources.

1) *Participation*. Decisions to limit care should be made by procedures and bodies that involve members of the general public, that is current and prospective patients, as well as administrators, physicians and other health professionals. Participation is important for several reasons. First, patients bear the principal consequences of specific rationing decisions and limitations on treatment, and so they should have input into what those limitations will be. Second, the public may have significantly different perspectives on the relative importance of different services and resource uses than health plan administrators, physicians and other health professionals; the public and patient perspectives should be a part of the decision-making process. Third, just as democratic legitimacy in the broader political process depends on the 'consent of the governed', here too the legitimacy of rationing decisions depends on the appropriate consent of those who will be governed by them.

2) *Openness and publicity*. The decision-making processes that set rationing limits need to be public and open to all persons affected by them; the transparency of decision-making is necessary to its legitimacy and public acceptance. Beyond simple openness and publicity about what rationing limits have been adopted, it is also necessary that the reasons for particular decisions to limit available care be publicly articulated and stated. This is important, in part, just because we do not have widely agreed-upon standards for making rationing decisions; publicly articulating the reasons for these decisions allows those reasons to be publicly discussed, accepted, challenged or revised. The goal is that through this process, over time, a set of rationing standards and principles will be developed which have been subject to public and professional scrutiny, similar to the way case law develops, over time, a set of standards in various areas of the law. Reasons for rationing decisions must also be given because what the reasons are for a particular limitation on available treatment partly determine its legitimacy: for example, not providing a particular treatment for some condition might

be justified in order to meet more urgent health needs of other patients, but not because the latter have a more effective or better politically connected advocacy group. It is not possible to assess the legitimacy of a particular limitation on beneficial care without knowing the reasons that limit has been adopted, and of course there is no reason to assume the legitimacy of any particular limit without having been offered the reasons for it.

3) *Independent appeals procedures*. There will often be reasonable disagreement or controversy about both general limitations of particular services that will be available on the NHS, as well as denials of particular services to particular patients. For those who are adversely affected by such decisions, and who reasonably believe them to be mistaken, it is important to have an appeals procedure that is independent of the decision-making body that determines the limits. The exact form of the appeals process that would make it independent of the decision-making body will obviously depend on the nature of the decision-making body itself, but the general point is that the appeals process must not be in any substantial way beholden to the decision-making body that sets the limits that are being appealed against. It is important that this appeals body be made available to patients, family members, physicians and other health care professionals, and health administrators, since any of these people may have a legitimate concern with decisions to limit beneficial care.

4) *Disclosure*. Patients should be informed about treatments, or other health care services with significant potential benefits for them, that are not available to them on the NHS because of rationing decisions that have been made. There are serious barriers to realising this full disclosure. In the USA, many managed care plans have so called 'gag rules' which forbid physicians to provide information to patients about care not available to them within the managed care plan, often on the justification that such limits are proprietary information. But, even without such legal restrictions on this disclosure, there is often a natural reluctance to inform patients about care that they might reasonably want, but that will not be available to them. In a study by Henry Aaron and William Schwartz carried out in the UK in the 1980s, when it was the practice not to dialyse patients with renal failure over the age of 60, they found that physicians tended to tell patients who were too old to qualify for renal dialysis that there was nothing more that could be done for them.[4] This implied that there was no further treatment that would benefit them, whereas in fact the truth was that a rationing decision had been made, even if informally, not to provide

treatment to such patients. The practice illustrates the difficulty and natural reluctance to be fully open with patients about the impact of rationing choices on them, but if patients are to have warranted trust in their physicians' commitments to their well-being then such openness is necessary. Some might object that it seems only cruel to tell patients about care from which they might benefit, but which will not be available to them within the NHS because of rationing decisions. But, even besides the need to avoid deception and maintain trust, patients may make important use of this information: for example, they may seek to utilise independent appeals procedures which should be available to them, or seek care elsewhere, or pay for it out-of-pocket.

How these various principles, and no doubt others as well, are operationalised in practice will depend on the detailed institutional structures within which they are applied, and I cannot pursue those details here. But these principles are necessary, in my view, to properly balance individual choice against equity and fair resource limits for health care. They reflect the fact that we lack substantive agreement on detailed standards for equitable rationing decisions and so must rely to a significant degree on fair procedures for making those decisions. Individuals cannot have unlimited choice in the services available to them in the NHS or any other health care system, but they can have assurance that their choices have been limited in fair ways that respect their interests and perspectives.

References

1   Brock D W, Daniels N. Ethical foundations of the Clinton Administration's proposed new health care system. *Journal of the American Medical Association* 1994; 271: 1189–96.

2   Brock D W. The ideal of shared decision-making between physicians and patients. In: *Life and Death: philosophical essays in biomedical ethics*. Cambridge: Cambridge University Press, 1993.

3   Daniels N, Sabin J. Limits to health care: fair procedures, democratic deliberation, and the legitimacy problem for insurers. *Philosophy and Public Affairs* 1997; 26: 303–50.

4   Aaron H J, Schwartz W B. *The Painful Prescription: rationing hospital care*. Washington, DC: The Brookings Institution, 1984.

Chapter 11

Managing disappointment in health care: three stories from the USA

James E Sabin and Norman Daniels*

For anyone reflecting on the values that should guide health care systems, the USA and the UK are like the contrasting principles of Yin and Yang. The US approach to health care is founded on the value of individual responsibility and a strong national preference for addressing problems through markets rather than government. Government's role is largely limited to providing a safety net for those who cannot participate effectively in the individualistic, competitive market arena. The UK approach is founded on values of social justice. Health care should be available to all, based only on need. The Government takes the central role in the funding and administration of the system. What can these moral antitheses learn from each other?

The key lessons for the USA to take from the UK are painfully obvious – universal access, the principle of solidarity and a robust general practice sector. But to those who have come of age supported by a national health service based on social justice ideals, it may seem presumptuous or even offensive to suggest that the UK could learn anything about health care values from the USA. We believe, however, that as counterintuitive as it might seem, the UK and the NHS can indeed derive useful lessons from the USA.

Paradoxically, the fact that the overarching US health care system is so glaringly unjust has led the best organisations within that unjust system to search for ways to create local or organisational justice within the sphere of their own control. For the past ten years, we have been studying these exemplary enterprises with a single core question in mind – how can health care organisations set priorities and limits that are clinically informed, ethically justifiable and politically acceptable? Put differently, how can health systems, whether Health Maintenance Organizations (HMOs) in the USA or health authorities in the UK, manage resource allocation in a way that constituents see as legitimate and fair?

* Please direct correspondence to Dr. Sabin at: Jim_Sabin@HPHC.org; or, HPHC – Department of Ambulatory Care and Prevention, 133 Brookline Avenue (6th floor), Boston MA 02215; Tel: 617-509-9926/Fax: 617-859-8112.

Legitimacy refers to the conditions under which moral authority over resource allocation decisions should be placed in the hands of private organisations (e.g. US health plans) or public agencies (e.g. UK health authorities). Fairness refers to the conditions under which patients, clinicians and the public have sufficient reason to accept a disappointing public or private resource allocation decision as fair. Legitimacy and fairness are distinctive issues. A legitimate authority can act unfairly, and an illegitimate one can deliver fair decisions. The issue at stake is not just *who* makes a decision but *how* the decision is made.

The essential lesson we have drawn from studies of mental health care, cancer treatment, decisions about new technologies, and insurance coverage for pharmaceuticals, is that to gain acceptance as legitimate and fair, organisations must hold themselves accountable for the reasonableness of their resource allocation policies.[1] In health care, 'reasonable' organisational policies are those that seek to reconcile the needs of individuals and the population the organisation serves. It is not enough for organisational policies to be reasonable – the rationales for these policies must also be 'transparent' or readily available to all of the concerned stakeholders. And, since even the wisest of policies may not apply to a particular patient or may need modification over time, accountability for reasonableness also requires that policies are subject to appeal and revision. Reasonable organisations learn, change and grow from their experience.

Fair-minded people may disagree about how to weigh the needs of individual patients and the totality of an insured population in making a particular decision or policy. But any health care system that pools funds to provide care for individuals as part of an insured population must seek that balance if it hopes to be seen as legitimate and fair.

At the level of fundamental health care values, accountability for reasonableness is a moral orientation that evinces respect and concern for the population being served. For organisations it is the population-level equivalent of what caring, respectful clinicians do to cultivate collaborative, trusting relationships with their patients. Patients care deeply about the attitudes, values and character of their clinicians. If they believe the clinician's heart is in the right place, treatments actually work better and they can forgive the inevitable disappointments that occur in every relationship. Metaphorically, organisational accountability for reasonableness corresponds to attitudes, values and character in the individual clinician.

At the level of pragmatic problem solving, accountability for reasonableness represents a way of dealing with value conflicts. The UK, like the USA, is a pluralistic society, with no widely shared values that could tell a health authority whether new funds should be invested in cancer care, improved mental health services, programmes for children or some combination of these factors. These are all worthy goals, but not all can be fully funded. In circumstances like this, where values conflict, accountability for reasonableness calls for resolution through a deliberative process. It specifies that the process should be accessible to the public, draw on relevant reasons (the needs of individuals and of the population), make its rationales as well as its conclusions widely available, and seek to improve its practices and policies over time by responding to appeals, calls for revision, and other opportunities for learning.

Embracing accountability for reasonableness is not simply a matter of establishing a policy or writing a mission statement – it must become a central component of organisational culture. As such it must be reflected in the behaviour and attitudes of staff, as well as in the policies and practices of the organisation. Anyone who has worked in or been served by an organisation committed to being accountable and reasonable knows what this means.

In the next three sections we describe how health organisations in the USA cultivate accountability for reasonableness. Although the mixed US system – with its primary reliance on a competitive market – and the NHS are very different, illness, fear, mortality and the need to make choices are the same in both settings. The aim of these 'stories' is to convey a deeper understanding of accountability for reasonableness by showing how exemplary US organisations seek to articulate their own core values and put those values into action in an accountable manner.

Making policy about Viagra

When the US Food and Drug Administration approved Viagra in February 1998, Harvard Pilgrim Health Care, an HMO that included drugs in its coverage, established an *ad hoc* working group to recommend policy for coverage of Viagra. That policy could range from a decision not to cover Viagra to coverage without any limits.

Like health authorities, US HMOs purchase health care for a specified population. The population of an HMO, however, is not defined by geography (residents of the district) but by enrollment. Most working Americans get health insurance through their employers. Harvard Pilgrim has contracts with thousands of employers in New England who offer the programme either as a single option or one of a series of choices. Many of the non-working poor have health insurance through a publicly supported programme (Medicaid) and can use that insurance to join Harvard Pilgrim if they wish. The over-65 population is covered by another public programme (Medicare) and can also choose Harvard Pilgrim for their insurance.

At the time of the Viagra debate, Harvard Pilgrim insured approximately 1 million members. Whereas health authorities get their budgets through legislative decisions, an HMO's budget is created by the insurance premiums paid into it on behalf of the members (and by those members who paid for their own insurance or were required by their employers to share part of the cost).

The group charged with recommending policy for coverage of Viagra debated whether Harvard Pilgrim should pay for the drug. Should Viagra be regarded as a 'treatment' to be covered like medications for asthma, diabetes or migraines, or should it be seen as an 'enhancement' or 'lifestyle' drug and not be covered at all, in the same way that cosmetic surgery is not covered? The planning group recognised that making policy about Viagra required addressing important values questions. And, at $7 per pill, with the potential for substantial demand, important cost-management questions were involved as well. They elected to consult with the Harvard Pilgrim Ethics Advisory Group.

The Ethics Advisory Group plays a significant role in Harvard Pilgrim's effort to be accountable for the reasonableness of its policies and practices. The Group includes members of the constituencies that are most concerned with the Harvard Pilgrim programme – consumers who are insured by the organisation, physicians who provide care under the insurance, employers who purchase Harvard Pilgrim insurance for their employees, and staff of the organisation. The Ethics Advisory Group deliberates about cases brought for consultation and offers non-binding advice about the ethical dimensions of the situation.

At the meeting, several participants applied terms like 'enhancement' and 'lifestyle drug' to Viagra and questioned whether it should be covered. The drift of their comments pointed to a potential rationale for not covering Viagra. At this point, a female member from an employer group that provided Harvard Pilgrim insurance for its employees spoke with great force. 'I can't believe that at the end of the 20th century – after all that Freud taught us – that we are talking as if sexuality were an optional matter of "lifestyle". Sex is an essential aspect of our being. To reduce the ability to have intercourse to the status of a "life-enhancing" activity is to belittle a patient's valid desire to restore a basic function.'

Her comments galvanised the Ethics Advisory Group into viewing Viagra as an innovation that offered real benefit and should not be dismissed as 'mere enhancement' or a 'lifestyle choice'. The Group, however, recognised organisational concerns about cost as valid. It advised Harvard Pilgrim's management that although Viagra should be allowed to compete for coverage within the overall budget of the organisation and should not be denigrated as 'mere enhancement', the fact that it offered benefit did not automatically mean that there were adequate funds available to pay for it. The value of adding coverage for Viagra had to be compared to the value provided by alternative uses of the funds. But the group advised in very strong terms that insofar as limits were put onto coverage for Viagra because of cost, the organisation should acknowledge the cost factor openly and clearly to members of the health plan and the public. Insofar as the NHS is expected to provide any treatment that is truly beneficial, this kind of acknowledgment would be more difficult in the UK.

In the aftermath of the Ethics Advisory Group discussion, Harvard Pilgrim decided to cover four Viagra pills a month at the discretion of the prescribing physician. Viagra was a very newsworthy topic in 1998, and the organisation's policy drew extensive attention from the regional media. Here is how the Medical Director discussed the policy with the press:

> I don't want to be in the position of saying how often people should have intercourse. We are not telling physicians they can write prescriptions for only four pills. They can write for 30 or 90 or whatever. What we are saying is that we will pay for only four a month. (Boston Globe 6/12/98 p c3)

> As to why Harvard Pilgrim settled on four pills as opposed to, say, eight, Dorsey [the Medical Director] admits there is no scientific logic to that number. 'It demonstrates a commitment to using the resource pool to help make it possible for people to use the medication … but it also reflects the fact that Viagra is too expensive for us to pay for unlimited use.' (Boston Globe 6/12/98 p c3)

Here is how the Medical Director addressed the question of whether Viagra should be seen as a 'lifestyle' or 'quality-of-life' drug:

What's 'quality of life' to one person might be 'absolutely essential' to somebody else. (Boston Herald 6/12/98 p 37)

Comparing the draft of a memo that was circulated to physicians who care for patients insured by Harvard Pilgrim to the final version is especially interesting in showing the Medical Director's determination to be explicit about the reasons behind the coverage policy.

Draft: *The expense of this product **also** played a part in the coverage decisions ... Paying for an unlimited number of Viagra tablets would divert [limited resources] away from **medically necessary, lifesaving** medications.* (Emphasis added)

This draft, written by a staff member, conjures up a vision of depriving a patient with cancer of curative treatment to provide 'unlimited' intercourse for a man with erectile dysfunction. Here is the Medical Director's version:

Final: *The expense of this product played a **major** part in the coverage decision ... Paying for an unlimited number of Viagra tablets would divert [limited resources] away from **other** uses.* (Emphasis added)

In shifting from 'expense ... also played a part' to 'expense ... played a major part', the Medical Director was using his bully pulpit to explain and teach. And by dropping reference to 'lifesaving' treatments he was conveying that there is a hierarchy of choices to be made, not a dichotomy between 'medically necessary, lifesaving' treatments and optional treatments. Viagra is a beneficial treatment but, even in a country as wealthy as the USA, not every beneficial treatment can be provided.

Managed care and HMOs are typically vilified in the US press, so the editorial response of Boston's major newspaper was not at all typical. In an editorial called 'A Sensible Compromise on Viagra', the *Boston Globe* wrote that 'Massachusetts HMOs have devised a policy that reasonably balances medical and cost considerations' (6/28/98, p a/19). This story about Harvard Pilgrim Health Care and Viagra policy suggests that with honest, articulate, educative leadership the public can understand the need to make difficult choices and accept limits as disappointing but fair.

Developing a culture of accountability

In the USA, management gurus preach the importance of clarity about mission and vision for organisational success. In response, organisations large and small have devoted substantial effort to crafting mission and vision statements. Almost every health organisation we are aware of includes some form of reference to 'consumers' (the most widely used term in US health policy circles for users of health care) in their statements of basic organisational values, as in 'consumer orientation,' 'consumer service' or 'consumer satisfaction'. The public, however, is sceptical – are these statements meaningful, or simply public relations fluff?

We have recently begun to study the ways in which exemplary health organisations try to implement their commitment to being accountable to consumers for the reasonableness of their policies and practices. One of our main study sites is the public mental health programme in Massachusetts. In the USA, federal, state and local government have traditionally played a major role in paying for mental health care, especially for the poor (who, even if they are employed, often do not have health insurance from their employers) and for those with serious and persisting mental illnesses. In Massachusetts, the public agencies responsible for this population are the Division of Medical Assistance (Medicaid) and the Department of Mental Health. On the basis of their belief that an experienced, private organisation would bring distinctive managerial skills and data management capacities to the job, the two departments hired a for-profit managed care company to purchase and manage mental health services for the population other than the services directly provided by the state. That company, the Massachusetts Behavioral Health Partnership (MBHP), has been the site of our study in Massachusetts.

In democratic systems, power resides with the people, who characteristically exercise their power through elected representatives. When these representatives vote to enact laws and policies, they confer legitimacy by giving their consent, and through them, the consent of the governed. It seems an easy – but erroneous – step of logic to infer that consumer participation contributes to legitimacy in health care in the same way – through representation and consent.

When consumers actually govern a health care organisation, representation and consent may indeed confer legitimacy on limit-setting policies. But true consumer governance is rare. In the USA, the Group Health Cooperative in

Washington state, in which consumer members of the Cooperative elect a consumer board of directors, is unique for size (600,000 members) and longevity (54 years) among consumer-governed programmes. In the vast majority of current health care settings, however, representation and consent do not apply with any literalness. For most health organisations, consumers are not elected to the roles they serve and the roles themselves are typically advisory, not governance.

But if representation and consent do not apply in a strict sense, does that mean that consumer participation can only be a sham? We think not. Our study of organisations like MBHP has convinced us that consumer participation plays a vital role in achieving legitimacy, but by improving accountability for reasonableness, not through representation or consent. Consumer participation is crucial to the three key elements of accountability for reasonableness: *transparency* regarding organisational policies and decisions; *deliberation* that properly recognises both individual and population needs; and the organisation's *capacity to learn from experience*, especially from criticism and appeals.[2]

Transparency

The enraged response of the US public and medical profession to managed care is due in significant degree to their perception that the explanations they are given for controversial policies and practices are not the real reasons. One often hears phrases like 'managed care is a black box' or 'managed care is about cost, not care'. When stakeholders believe they are being kept in the dark about crucial aspects of a fundamental good like health care, they fill in the blanks by imagining the worst.

It is important to distinguish between the bureaucratic concept of 'disclosure', which can be satisfied legalistically by arcane phrases hidden in the fine print of long documents, and 'transparency', which connotes open and free exchange. The Massachusetts programme cultivates transparency by involving consumers at multiple points of the management process – through a Consumer Advisory Council that meets monthly, a Consumer Satisfaction Team in which consumers interview patients to get their views about their treatment, *ad hoc* task forces, and an open-door policy at both the public purchaser and the Massachusetts Behavioral Health Partnership. 'Disclosure' is a one-time bureaucratic event. 'Transparency' is a relationship and an ongoing process.

Deliberation

Simply 'listening' to what consumers say does not create legitimacy. To be meaningful, consumer voice must make a difference in what organisations do and ultimately in the health outcomes that are achieved. Consumers rightfully become cynical about organisations that claim to 'listen' without taking action. The situation is complicated, however, because valuing consumer participation cannot mean 'agreeing', since the values put forward by other stakeholders must be considered as well. Consumer views are always important but they are not always correct.

MBHP cultivates a consumer role in deliberation by including consumers in key policy-making activities in an ongoing manner. Thus, in developing annual performance standards for the programme, members of the Consumer Advisory Council deliberate about their own top priorities for the year, after which they join with clinicians, programme managers and other stakeholders to integrate the different perspectives. Consumers reviewed and commented on all of the sixteen performance standards incorporated into the 2001 contract between MBHP and the state agencies. Four of the 16 had been directly proposed by the Consumer Advisory Council. As an example, the Consumer Advisory Council emphasised the importance of enhancing consumer advocacy skills. This led to a performance standard requiring MBHP to develop a Consumer Leadership Academy 'to promote self-empowerment and recovery-oriented approaches'.

Organisational learning

Most US regulatory attention to improving managed care focuses on appeals and the opportunity to bring lawsuits, but these provide a very limited form of consumer voice, given national experience that consistently demonstrates limited use of appeals mechanisms, and the Dickensian slowness of the legal process. Meaningful consumer participation requires more than the kinds of appeals processes and right to sue that form the centerpiece of legislative and regulatory 'reform'.

Massachusetts cultivates the consumer role in organisational learning by ensuring that consumers have central formal and informal roles in a 'try it–fix it' approach to policy and practice. The Consumer Advisory Council regularly reviews reports on the status of performance standards. It makes recommendations about new programmes and how they should be developed. The independently incorporated Consumer Satisfaction Team conducts surveys of consumer satisfaction with services across the state. More than 25 consumer-led peer educator groups provide education and support for recovery, and also create the equivalent of consumer focus groups, the results of which are reported to the managed care organisation and the public purchaser at meetings, and informally. As an example, a series of critical anecdotes about emergency services led to a meeting among the managed care organisation, Division of Medical Assistance, Department of Mental Health, and activist members of the Alliance for the Mentally Ill, at which a series of problems were identified and an improvement strategy put into place.

The important aspects of the MBHP story are not the details of how consumers are involved in influencing policy and practice. Nothing the organisation does is rocket science. What matters is the day in, day out consistency of the organisation's interactions with consumers. MBHP and public agency leadership have open doors for consumers. Consumers participate in objective setting, programme evaluation and efforts to improve quality. The organisation provides excellent staff support for the consumer committees. US health plans or UK health authorities seek to cultivate accountability for reasonableness, then transparency, deliberation and organisational learning must be central components of everyday organisational life, not pieties written on paper.

Last-chance treatments – US approaches to the child B dilemma

The most difficult and explosive responsibility for any health care system is deciding whether patients with life-threatening illnesses will receive insurance coverage for unproven treatments they believe may make the difference between life and death.

Potentially life-saving treatments with proven efficacy and safety (proven net benefit), and quack treatments for which there is no scientific rationale, rarely pose major problems about insurance coverage. In countries as wealthy as the USA or UK, clearly effective last-chance treatments without alternatives generally are and should be covered virtually all the time. When shared resources from co-operative schemes are involved, as in public or private insurance or the NHS, as opposed to situations in which individuals pay with their own resources, quack treatments will and should virtually never be covered, even if the patient or doctor passionately believes in the purported cure.

Readers in the UK will recognise these issues as the core ethical questions debated openly in the Jaymee Bowen or 'child B' case. They are the kinds of decisions discussed so well for the NHS context by Chris Ham and colleagues.[3]

This third story from the USA focuses on how two large organisations – the Aetna insurance company and Kaiser Permanente – have dealt with ethical issues of the kind involved in situations like that of child B.

Deciding about promising but unproven last-chance treatments requires consideration of at least four distinctive values:

- First, virtually all societies agree that *some* priority should be given to the urgent claims of patients in last-chance situations. The difficult challenge is to decide *how much* priority should be given in the particular patient's situation.

- Second, since the contested treatments are typically very expensive, the organisation's (or health authority's) responsibility for providing responsible stewardship of collective resources comes into play.

- Third, if unproven treatments are provided before they have been studied scientifically, the public good of scientific knowledge is threatened, and we may be delayed in learning that a treatment is ineffective or even harmful. In the USA, well-intentioned but misguided legislatures and courts began to require coverage of stem-cell transplant for metastatic breast cancer in the early 1990s. The treatment was consequently widely applied before research showed that it does not improve survival.

- Finally, respect for the individual patient and family (patient 'autonomy') means inviting participation in collaborative decision-making about the risks and benefits of the proposed treatment.

Urgency, stewardship, scientific knowledge and patient autonomy are all positive values. The challenge is deciding how much weight to give to each in situations in which different participants may assess the relative importance of the values differently.

In 1991, the television programme *60 Minutes* featured a story about the Aetna insurance company declining coverage for bone marrow transplant for breast cancer. Aetna responded by developing a new programme, in which when state-based medical directors (similar to public health directors in health authorities) received a request for an unproven but promising last-chance cancer treatment that was not covered under established Aetna policy, they referred the request to the company's head office in Connecticut, where a consulting oncologist reviewed the clinical situation. A key feature of the programme was that the head office oncologist was only empowered to approve requests. If the consulting oncologist believed that the request did not represent reasonable clinical practice for the particular patient, the case was automatically referred to the Medical Care Ombudsman Program.[4]

The Ombudsman Program, which was founded in 1991, provides independent expert opinion about serious but ambiguous clinical situations. On a timetable that can be as short as 24 hours, the Ombudsman Program will put together a panel of up to three experts, with no affiliation to the insurer or the provider of the proposed treatment, to assess whether the proposed treatment has any scientific rationale for the particular patient. Typically, at least one of the experts is prepared to testify in court if the case should come to litigation.

Aetna did not restrict its own consulting oncologist from rendering negative coverage decisions because the consultant lacked competence. The problem Aetna was trying to solve with its last-chance programme was one of trust, not lack of technical expertise. The fact and appearance of conflict of interest was removed. If Aetna would say no only if an independent consultant said no, then the 'no' should not be construed as a cost-driven decision. In circumstances of life-threatening illness and ambiguous information, the patient and family's trust in the decision-making process can be the difference between peace and outrage, or acceptance versus litigation.

In 1993, the Northern California region of the Kaiser Permanente HMO took the programme that Aetna had developed in an insurance context and adapted it for its own 3600-physician pre-paid group practice. As a not-for-profit organisation providing medical care to a defined population, Kaiser Permanente has much in common with health authorities in the NHS.

Like Aetna, Northern California Kaiser Permanente decided to let patients in last-chance situations know that they could go outside of Kaiser for an independent opinion from the Ombudsman Program if they were not satisfied with the internal decision-making process. This was a controversial step for Kaiser to take. Some Kaiser doctors worried that allowing automatic appeal outside of the HMO would unleash a costly flood of external appeals and diminish the group's ability to manage care rationally.

What actually happened was exactly the opposite. From 1994 to 1996, only six of the 2.5 million northern California members asked for referral to the Ombudsman Program. When patient and family concerns about Kaiser's trustworthiness and potential conflicts of interest were addressed in advance by the option of going outside of Kaiser for a binding independent consultation, they were much readier to enter into a reflective dialogue with their Kaiser physicians about what treatment approach really made sense for them.

The story about Aetna and Kaiser Permanente would appear to teach a suggestive moral lesson. If a promising, but unproven, last-chance treatment is viewed by acknowledged experts as the most appropriate treatment for the patient, and if the patient understands the risks, then organisations have no better option than to rely on the informed decision of patients and their clinicians. This is not the same as saying that a patient can be granted just any last wish regarding treatment. There must be some basis in evidence and expert view that the therapy is not quackery. In the external review model adopted by Aetna and Kaiser Permanente, that expert view is provided by the independent panel. Under those conditions, simply refusing to provide coverage would fail to acknowledge the obligation not to impose paternalistically a plan's (or health authority's) own judgement about acceptable risks and benefits on the choices of desperately ill patients with few options. To be sure, the organisation's role as guardian of shared resources is reduced, but this is defensible in light of the urgency of the patient's needs, and the special importance, in light of the uncertainty and the severity of need, of promoting a climate of shared decision-making.

Given the high emotional and monetary cost of public controversy about contested decisions, a proponent of the Aetna/Kaiser approach might argue that the decision to hold to a hard-line denial of coverage is so likely to lead to a waste of resources that the more efficient way to respect resource limits is to adopt the more lenient-seeming strategy towards last-chance therapies. The Ombudsman Program recommends against approximately half of the proposed therapies. The fact that only ten cases per thousand denials have gone to court suggests that the process of independent expert review may enhance responsible stewardship.

Conclusion

With regard to values, the USA and UK are pluralistic societies and are becoming more so over time. The hope for a single shared ranking of values for health care is quixotic. Health authorities in the NHS and HMOs in the USA require fair and accepted processes for making decisions and policies.

The current US health care system has engendered an extraordinarily high level of distrust. Readers in the UK can get a sense of the environment by viewing two US movies. In *As Good as it Gets*, audiences cheered when Helen

Hunt, playing the mother of a child with asthma, lambasts her HMO for paying more attention to the bottom line than to her son's medical needs. In *The Rainmaker*, an insurance company is engaged in a criminal conspiracy to collect premiums while paying no health care claims at all! Like animals or plants living in a hostile climate, exemplary US organisations have devoted extraordinary effort to creating local conditions for legitimacy and trust. It is at the level of the organisation – not the global system – that potentially useful lessons about values can be derived for the NHS.

We believe that the essence of these lessons is the importance of accountability for reasonableness – transparency, deliberation and the capacity to learn from experience. While we originally thought of accountability for reasonableness primarily as a characterisation of fair decision-making process, we have come to see it as a fundamental value in itself, analogous to 'character' or 'virtue' in the individual clinician, especially the virtues of fairness, integrity and care.

The story about coverage for Viagra at Harvard Pilgrim Health Care shows what the abstract concept of 'transparency' can look like in action. The organisation's willingness to be open about the role of cost in Viagra policy allowed it to acknowledge the benefits the drug provides, rather than denigrating it as 'mere enhancement' as a way of rationalising a policy of limited coverage. As a beneficial but not life-and-death technology, Viagra offers opportunities for public debate and learning, in ways that are different from emergency situations like child B or the cases discussed by Ham and McIver.[5] Important but non-crisis decisions like Viagra policy are especially important for long-range learning about using limited resources fairly.

The story about the Massachusetts Behavioral Health Partnership offers a humble but important lesson. It illustrates how the organisational 'character' component of accountability for reasonableness emerges from consistent, undramatic ways of working with consumers and the public over time. Cases like that of child B explode into public awareness in a riveting manner. Studies like *Tragic Choices in Health Care*[6] provide crucial learning opportunities for organisations and health professionals. But on the basis of all that is known about how collaborative, trusting clinical relationships evolve over time, we believe that the small, recurrent patterns of accountability, as practised by organisations such as MBHP, can also enhance public learning and foster legitimacy.

Finally, the story about how Aetna and Kaiser Permanente have dealt with controversial last-chance treatments suggests that a process like access to independent experts as a means of resolving contested last-chance decisions can help patients and families reach mutually acceptable conclusions with their clinicians and health plans. In the USA, there has been an emerging consensus that these last-chance decisions cannot be determined by general policies but must be made patient by patient. However, with disciplined attention to the principles embedded in a series of 'one of a kind' decisions, an analogue to legal precedent and case law begins to emerge.

In the USA, these precedents indicate that patients, families and the public can accept tragic choices much more readily when there has been prompt, undefensive movement to consultation with an independent panel before a crisis of distrust has erupted. The precedents further suggest that in circumstances of great need, but unestablished efficacy, any treatment that is provided should be done in a context that promotes further learning about efficacy – especially a clinical trial if one is available. There is as yet no explicit consensus about what counts as adequate evidence of efficacy in the absence of controlled trials, but there is broad acceptance of the mechanism of using independent experts who are asked to recommend the right treatment for an individual patient as a surrogate for adequate evidence.

The UK and the NHS have stimulated an important international debate about the relative merits of explicit and implicit approaches to limit-setting. We believe that the experience of exemplary health organisations in the USA – struggling to achieve legitimacy and to set limits fairly in an unjust health care system – points the way to a middle path. Like explicit approaches to limit-setting, accountability for reasonableness calls for open deliberation in which the rationale for policy decisions is presented in a transparent manner. Unlike explicit limit-setting, however, it does not start from a pre-existing ethical framework that specifies how competing values should be ranked. Like implicit approaches to limit-setting, accountability for reasonableness emphasises the importance of a process that focuses on the particularities of case at hand, but unlike implicit limit-setting it makes extensive use of the 'case law' provided by previous policies and decisions.

An ethic that emphasises the crucial importance of fair process and calls for development of ethical guidance on the basis of precedent could come to grief on the basis of different conclusions in different US organisations or UK health authorities. Even if the different conclusions arise from justifiable but differing weights being given to the relevant values, this will be difficult for participants in decision-making and the public to understand. This makes learning that crosses organisational or geographical boundaries especially important. The learning network on priority setting coordinated by the Health Services Management Centre at the University of Birmingham and the multi-organisational Harvard Medical School/National Institute of Health 'BEST' (Best Ethical STrategies for managed care) project exemplify what needs to be done.[7]

The authors thank the Greenwall Foundation and the Open Society Institute Program on Medicine as a Profession for their generous support.

References

1   Daniels N, Sabin J E. The ethics of accountability and the reform of managed care organizations. *Health Affairs* 1998; 17: 50–69; and Daniels N, Sabin J E. *Setting Limits Fairly: can we learn to share medical resources?* New York: Oxford University Press, in press.

2   Daniels N, Sabin J E. Limits to health care: fair procedures, democratic deliberation, and the legitimacy problem for insurers. *Philosophy and Public Affairs* 1997; 26: 303–50.

3   Ham C, Pickard S. *Tragic Choices in Health Care: the case of child B.* London: King's Fund, 1998; and Ham C, McIver S. *Contested Decisions: priority setting in the NHS.* London: King's Fund, 2000.

4   Medical Care Management Corporation. *Medical Care Ombudsman Program.* www.mcman.com/493brochure.htm, 2001.

5   Ham and McIver, 2000, above.

6   Ham and Pickard, 1998, above.

7   Ham and McIver, 2000, above, p.3; and Randel L, Pearson S, Sabin J E *et al.* How managed care can be ethical. *Health Affairs* 2001; 20: 43–56.

Chapter 12

Caring for strangers: solidarity, diversity and the NHS*

Alan Wolfe and Jytte Klausen

For the 100 years preceding the 1970s, progressives in Europe and the USA pursued a politics of solidarity. The Left demanded the creation and expansion of the welfare state. Public policy should redistribute income, and subsidise, if not deliver directly, essential services such as education and, especially, health. The ideal was a society in which the inequalities associated with social class would fade away.

That ideal remains in place, but from the 1970s onwards it has been gradually eclipsed by another ideal – the promotion of diversity. Groups that once experienced discrimination would now be accorded recognition. The plethora of languages and cultures created by immigration and the greater tolerance of domestic minority groups, such as gay people, would be celebrated in the name of multiculturalism, not trampled in the name of assimilation. Because different groups have different values and understandings of right and wrong, the state would have to be neutral between them. The good society became one in which no person would have to live with a sense of shame because his or her gender, race, sexuality or able-bodied status is different from the majority's.

Herein lies the progressive dilemma of the 21st century. Solidarity and diversity are both desirable objectives. Unfortunately, they can also conflict. A sense of solidarity creates a readiness to share with strangers, which in turn underpins a thriving welfare state. But it is easier to feel solidarity with those who broadly share one's own values and way of life. Modern progressives committed to diversity often fail to acknowledge this. They employ an over-abstract and unrealistic notion of affinity, implying that we ought to have the same feelings of generosity or solidarity towards a refugee from the other side of the world as we do towards our next-door neighbour.

---

* This is a revised version of our article, 'Other People', which appeared in the December 2000 issue of *Prospect* magazine; www.prospect-magazine.co.uk. The King's Fund would like to thank *Prospect* for permission to reprint an amended version of that article.

These difficulties, great enough in dealing with the welfare state in general, are of special relevance when the welfare state concerns itself with health. For one thing, disease and health vary from one ethnic group to another. According to the 1999 *Health Survey for England*, Pakistani and Bangladeshi men and women reported worse overall health conditions than the general population, while Chinese men and women reported better health.[2] Second, some diseases disproportionately affect certain ethnic groups, even when controlling for income, age and socio-economic status. The incidence of heart conditions (angina and heart attacks) was nearly double that of the general population among Bangladeshi men and only one-third among black Caribbean and Chinese men. Even a phenomenon that might, at first glance, appear to be culturally neutral, such as the occurrence of major and minor accidents, was found by the *Health Survey* to vary by ethnic group. Many diseases are not directly related to lifestyle, but some of the diseases that, because of their prevalence are particularly important from a public health perspective, such as diabetes, obesity and alcoholism, are directly related to lifestyle and, hence, also culture.

In addition, questions of prevention and treatment inevitably intersect with questions of culture. The best way to prevent diseases of the liver is to control alcohol consumption, but some ethnic groups encourage drinking while others shun it. Much the same is true of tobacco and its associated risk of lung cancer. Complications from pregnancy vary with the number of pregnancies, and that in turn varies with the attitudes toward birth control among different cultures. Rates of HIV transmission are overwhelmingly influenced by sexual behaviours and incidence of drug addiction, and both of those factors vary depending on culture and lifestyle. The same could be said about risks associated with abortion. As we learn more about disease, we learn more about their environmental causes, and within the range of environmental factors are not just physical conditions like air quality but social conditions like propensities toward safe or unsafe practices.

Finally, culture matters in the very ways in which we think about health and disease, including the ways in which we collect data about them. If a particular group in the population is at risk for a specific condition, is it the obligation of government to publicise the relevant statistics in a way designed to enhance prevention? Or would such publication – by, for example, demonstrating an association between disease and a practice that, such as drug addiction, could be taken as a negative stereotype – contribute to racism? The fact that we know so much more about conditions that can be associated with disease, however positive from a public health point of view, is not always positive in what we learn about those conditions. An example is provided by the recent efforts of the Blair government to encourage 'ethnic monitoring' audits of how effective public intervention, such as drug prevention or health and social services, can be in specific ethnic communities. Such efforts may be used to argue for additional resources to address specific needs. They may also reveal information about variations in lifestyles and practices that raise difficult questions about responsibility and the allocation of costs.

In a society in which health care is primarily a matter of the market and individual choice, such as the USA, questions involving the relationship between culture and health, while important, are kept largely out of public debate. But in a society such as the UK, which has made a commitment to creating and maintaining a national health service, such questions bring up to date and sharpen the dilemma between solidarity and diversity that has always been an issue when government assumes a major role in promoting particular values. Our purpose in this chapter is to review the historic conflict between solidarity and diversity in the British welfare state, to examine the form that this conflict takes today in a number of countries at a time of heightened concern with multiculturalism, and to suggest some possible implications this conflict of values may pose for the National Health Service (NHS).

Solidarity and diversity: a brief history

In the early days of the British welfare state, in the 1940s and 1950s, the conflict between solidarity and diversity was less prevalent than it is now. People believed that they were paying the social welfare part of their taxes to people rather like themselves who faced the same risks and problems. For most people, paying tax was a kind of enlightened self-interest. Just 25 years' later, Britain had become a much more diverse place. This was not just a matter of ethnic diversity. Rather, big differences in values began to emerge between (and within) the generations. It was also the beginning of the end of a long process of national homogenisation which had begun in the late 18th century and encompassed the creation of empire; the forging of new national institutions in the Victorian period; and the two world wars of the first half of the 20th century. Britishness – encapsulated in institutions such as the BBC and the NHS – was shot through with more particular regional and class identities, but it had become a powerful binding force. By the 1970s, that binding force began to weaken and it has been gradually unravelling ever since. In some instances this is welcome, but the price paid is a diminution in solidarity. It seems plausible to suggest, for example, that this weakening is one

factor behind the emergence in the 1970s of popular support for tax resistance
– if the ties that bind you to increasingly diverse fellow citizens are loosened,
you are likely to be less inclined to share your resources with them.

The great 19th-century theorists of progress, from John Stuart Mill to Karl
Marx, distrusted the claims of particularistic groups. And T H Marshall's essay,
'Citizenship and Social Class',[3] one of the founding documents of the modern
welfare state, posits an inevitable tension between social class, which is
particular, and citizenship, which is universal. Marshall is famous for
describing three kinds of citizenship rights: civil, political and social, each of
which are associated with a particular century, beginning with the 18th.
Citizenship rights, especially social ones, promoted what Marshall called 'class
abatement'. He accepted a certain amount of economic inequality as
inevitable. What he wanted eliminated was the badge of inferiority associated
with a class system as rigid as that of 19th-century Britain.

The theorists of the welfare state were unabashed nationalists. William
Beveridge, in his 1942 report,[4] recognised that a system of social insurance
would require 'a sense of national unity overriding the interests of any class or
section'. In a 1942 lecture,[5] he said: 'One of the weaknesses of many reformers
in the past is that they have not taken account of the immense feeling of
patriotism in the British people, or that loving pride which we have in our
country.' That was not just war-time rhetoric; the welfare state's
communitarianism predated the Second World War. In 1931, R H Tawney[6]
wrote that 'what a community requires … is a common culture, because,
without it, it is not a community at all'.

In contrast to Friedrich Hayek and other free-market theorists, Marshall and
Beveridge did not believe that an expansion of the state came at the expense of
individual freedom. On the contrary, government power and individual
capacity depended on each other. Government was required, not only to frame
new social policies, but to confront entrenched forces, such as class, which
prevented people from full participation in their society. The distrust that
welfare state theorists expressed toward particularism was the flip-side of the
faith they had in the state and social citizenship. Where the claims of class –
or, for that matter, race and religion – were weak, the state would need less
power. But because the social effects of class had been so deeply etched into
British life, the state would have to be strong in response.

The politics of diversity starts out with assumptions similar to the politics of
national solidarity: where we end up in life should not be dependent upon the

conditions into which we are born. But from that common starting point, theorists of diversity go on to posit relationships between individuals, groups and the state which are widely at odds with an earlier generation of welfare state advocates.

Proponents of identity politics argue that prejudices against women or racial minorities are so deep that it is naive to expect them to 'abate' in the near future. It therefore serves the cause of social justice to take groups, as well as individuals, into account. Individuals, after all, are not isolated neurons bouncing around in a scientist's cloud chamber; they are constituted by the language, ethnicity and gender of their birth; their outlook on the world is shaped by the world's outlook on them. So, supporters of identity politics attribute to groups many of the qualities that earlier liberal theorists attributed to people: they have consciousness, they have interests and, in a truly just society, they should have rights.

If groups within the nation state receive greater recognition, it must follow that conceptions of over-arching national solidarity must receive less. In the recent report sponsored by the Runnymede Trust, *The Future of Multi-Ethnic Britain*, Bhikhu Parekh – the report's co-ordinator – argues along exactly these lines.[7] The Parekh Report can be read in part as a response to an earlier Home Office document.[8] In language indebted to Marshall and Beveridge, the Home Office announced its commitment to creating '"One Nation" in which racial diversity would be celebrated', 'everyone recognises their responsibilities', and 'everyone is treated according to their needs and rights'. The Parekh Report is sceptical of the 'One Nation' idea and asks whether we can prevent it being 'oppressive or jingoistic'.

Beveridge may have spoken of the 'loving pride' he had in his country, but the Parekh Report famously states that 'Britishness, as much as Englishness, has systematic, largely unspoken, racial connotations'. National unity in the UK never existed, the Report argues, nor should it exist now; a 'fixed conception of national identity and culture' is the enemy of diversity and underpins racism. People living in the UK cannot adhere to 'the values of one community'. Such agreement as those living in the UK require in order to function as good neighbours can be provided by 'international human rights standards ... that form part of the moral dialogue in all parts of the world'.

The Parekh Report argues that in a multicultural world people have many identities, some overlapping, some competing. To uproot them from the particular groups which do so much to fashion their identity and turn them into citizens whose first loyalty must be to the nation state is to, potentially, deprive them of important cultural tools: their language, if it is different from the dominant one; their faith, if it is not Christian; their literature, if it is not represented in schools; their sense of self-worth, if society devalues their traditions. As Parekh once put the point in a discussion of the Rushdie affair,[9] Muslim immigrants in the UK 'did have an obligation to obey the laws of the land, but British society too had obligations to them … To insist that they and other minorities should accept the British way of life amounted to treating them as second-class citizens'. What Marshall and Beveridge saw as a precondition for a properly functioning welfare state Parekh views as domination. 'Immigrants owe loyalty to the British state,' he notes, 'but not to British values, customs, and way of life.'

The Parekh Report does talk about striking 'a balance between cohesion, equality and difference', but then proceeds to ignore the problem. Its recommendations amount to little more than an attempt to broaden the elite which administers the state. More money should be spent on non-English community leaders; minorities should be appointed in greater numbers to boards and commissions; there should be more non-whites in the media and the arts. Aside from demands for increased child allowances and support for asylum seekers, the Report seeks no substantial extra funds for social programmes.

Like nearly all advocates of diversity, Parekh is a man of the Left who thinks of himself as a friend of the welfare state. Yet welfare plays little or no role in the Report's conception of British society. It offers a history of Britain designed to demonstrate how arbitrary the idea of Britain has been. It highlights the break with Rome, the union of the Scottish and English crowns, and Irish incorporation. Absent from the list are the bombing of London and Coventry, and the 1945 reforms which established the modern welfare state. Except for a few controversial issues that we will examine shortly, the Parekh Report spends little time discussing the NHS, the creation of which most Britons would regard as a singular milestone in their history. The Report's history of the welfare state encompasses in one sentence three centuries of social reform, from the elimination of the Poor Laws to the outlawing of child labour. This is history through the wrong end of the telescope. Many Britons take pride in the welfare state's contemporary accomplishments, not in the nation's dim, often mythic, past.

But, the Report's biggest confusion is over whether the state has the right to impose Western, liberal values on minorities. This is a familiar conundrum for multiculturalists who are also liberals – and the Parekh Report fails to resolve it. The Report urges agreement on fundamental values, including 'the equal moral worth of all human beings'. But then it goes on to suggest that 'different individuals and communities should be free to lead their self-chosen lives'. 'Society may legitimately ban forced marriages,' it says, 'or those based on duress or deceit, but it should respect the custom in many cultures of basing marriages on introductions arranged by parents.' At one point, the Report seems to suggest that polygamy ought to be tolerated. Then, in a different mood, it states: 'It is legitimate to ban the unequal treatment of women even though this may enjoy cultural authority in certain communities.' The philosopher Susan Muller Okin recently asked whether multiculturalism was bad for women.[10] The preference the Report gives for immigrant ways of life suggests that it is.

In *Rethinking Multiculturalism*, Bhikhu Parekh argued that equality 'is inseparable and ontologically no more important than human differences'.[11] In other words, equality and diversity are both important and our attempts to balance the two depend upon a calculation of the trade-offs involved. This seems a reasonable approach, and in fact this is how policy-makers generally arrive at compromise solutions when faced with policy dilemmas. But the difficulties involved become apparent when we consider issues such as female circumcision, funeral pyres, or *sati*, the expectation that widows follow their husbands into death. Parekh argues that *sati* should be banned, but not from the perspective of the right to life or the dignity of life, which have informed declarations of basic rights such as the Charter of Fundamental Rights of the European Union (Article 2), passed in December 2000 at the Nice Summit meeting, or the 1948 UN Universal Declaration of Human Rights (Article 1). Parekh instead arrives at this conclusion by means of balancing the claims of tradition against the need to protect women who may or may not be in a position to make an informed decision. On balance, he concludes, it is best to ban the practice, although arguments could be made for making a 'conscientious exemption' for deeply religious women wishing to kill themselves, provided that their desire to do so is 'suitably ascertained by government officials'. (p.281) It is difficult to imagine that Britain, in the name of multiculturalism, should put the NHS to the task of issuing permits for self-immolation.

Burial practices are another example of immigrant practices that have strained Western societies. In Denmark, the creation of Muslim cemeteries has been held up for a decade due to a thicket of environmental regulations and zoning rules. At issue is the requirement that the dead cannot be disturbed. Danish burial plots are protected for 25 years. While it may be easy to agree that the Danes ought to show more flexibility in their application of land-use rules, Parekh's suggestion that Western government should set up 'closed and official designated places', where funeral pyres may be built and the ashes from the cremated scattered, conjures scenarios of environmental impact regulations and NIMBY (Not-In-My-Back-Yard) politics that only those who thrive on conflict would relish.

When does the balancing approach – what Parekh calls the 'dialogical' approach – break down? Principles, as well as calculations of cost, can get in the way quickly. Rights have costs, as Stephen Holmes and Cass Sunstein have suggested.[12] Multiculturalist theory tends to pay scant attention to either, but once we begin to translate multiculturalist ideas into practical policy they cannot be avoided. Multiculturalists have held up as an example of 'good' policy the legal exemptions for Sikhs who, for religious reasons, cannot wear helmets. (A 1972 law requiring all motorcyclists to wear helmet was amended in 1976 to exempt turban-wearing Sikhs. A similar exemption was made in 1989 to work-safety rules that require helmets on construction sites.) Parekh recommends the exemptions as examples of how respect for difference may be accommodated without violating the principle of equality (p.244). Parekh finds that the balancing requirement between respect for diversity and equality is satisfied because the costs of *additional* injuries – that is injuries that can be traced to the fact that the patient was not wearing a helmet – caused by wearing a turban in place of a helmet is carried by Sikhs relying on the exemptions. But it is exactly for this reason that the Sikh exemptions hardly provide a 'best practices' example for public health policies. The costs to the patients – rather than the tax-paying general public – is too high. The rule may work to exempt private parties from paying for damages to the life and limbs of a patient caused by the patient's lifestyle or cultural practices, but it hardly works to limit the obligations of the NHS in a similar fashion. Since diseases and health problems are related to lifestyles, how would we distinguish between health care costs incurred because of dietary habits (which multiculturalist argue should be recognised) or by other types of increased risk associated with cultural or religious practices? Parekh argues that the injured party – the turban-wearing Sikh – is personally responsible for the health cost incurred because of cultural practices. He neglects to consider that health insurance, albeit public, ultimately comes from private pockets, just as car insurance monies do. If we assume that he thinks that the NHS should carry the cost of accidents caused by observance of religious or cultural prohibitions, taxpayers obviously have a legitimate interest in regulating risky behaviour, much as they do in the case of smoking and obesity. Yet even under those circumstances, most health care workers would be more concerned about the direct bodily and financial costs to patients, rather than the highly diluted cost to taxpayers. In my view, Parekh forgets to consider that many cultural practices are harmful to people, Sikhs and Christians, and that is why health care professionals have worked to change them. Moreover, we find it risky politically to suggest that individuals are responsible for their own follies – be they the result of religious prohibitions or more vaguely defined cultural practices. Where do we draw the line between public and private responsibility in such cases? Smoking causes cancer. Should cancer patients, therefore, be held responsible for the cost of treatments directly related to their smoking habit, if they have been life-long smokers, despite having been told that their smoking poses a danger to their health? It has become practice to charge hikers who venture past signs posting warnings not to go further for the cost to public agencies of their rescue. The attempts on the part of US states to recover Medicare costs for treating smokers from US cigarette makers have already raised concerns that this is the first step towards off-loading public responsibilities for self-inflicted health problems.

In 1956, the sociologists Edward Shils and Michael Young wrote: 'Over the past century, British society, despite distinctions of nationality and social status, has achieved a degree of moral unity equalled by no other large national state ... constitutional monarchy and political democracy has played a part in the creation and maintenance of this moral consensus.'[13] Since that was written, the monarchy has become tarnished as a symbol of moral unity – its place, arguably, taken by the NHS – and the country has become far more diverse in values, lifestyle and ethnicity. There can be no return to that moral unity. But Marshall's ideas about citizenship matter more in this diverse and individualistic world than they did in the Britain that emerged out of the Second World War. It is when we are most different from each other that we most require agreement on what makes us common members of a society. Agreement to abide by the laws of the land is not enough. Of course the idea of 'Britishness' cannot be fixed (consider the way that the history of empire was taught 100 years ago and how it is taught now – reflecting not only the different faces in the classroom but changed attitudes towards race and violence). But this does not mean that we can afford to abandon the idea of 'Britishness'. The hard question is which values and symbols, which cultural and linguistic norms, are the minimum we require to achieve cohesion.

The USA, the UK and Scandinavia

The USA and Europe approach this argument from different places on the solidarity/diversity spectrum. Notwithstanding the USA's nationalism and the strength of its civic culture, it has – as an immigrant society – usually placed diversity above solidarity. This is one reason for the weakness of the US welfare state, and why the group most strongly committed to it, African-Americans, is also the most hostile to unrestricted immigration. But scepticism towards the state in the USA precludes a significant role for government in the management of social solidarity. The British Social Attitudes special international report of 1989 pointed out that only 36 per cent of Americans thought it was 'definitely the government's responsibility to provide health care for the sick', compared with 86 per cent of Britons. There were similar gulfs of 16 per cent (USA) to 45 per cent (UK) on providing a decent standard of living for the unemployed and 17 per cent to 48 per cent on reducing income differences between rich and poor.

In continental Europe, the stress on social solidarity, managed by the state, is even greater than in the individualistic UK. For reasons linked to feudalism, Christianity, and the fear of revolution or invasion, the idea of a benign national state protecting all its citizens is a powerful one – most famously embodied by French republicanism, assimilating citizens into a state religion that transcends class and ethnicity. But the historic preference for solidarity before diversity is now a source of great tension too. Nowhere is this truer than in the small, egalitarian, formerly ethnically homogeneous states of Sweden and Denmark.

The Governments in both these countries have issued reports along the lines of the Home Office's *Race Equality in Public Services*. Faced with the prospect of immigrants making up almost 20 per cent of the population within the next 20 years, Danes and Swedes have reasserted national values. The Swedes have embraced the idea of diversity but rejected multiculturalism; the Danes have rejected multiculturalism and barely accepted diversity at all. Yet those reports have been widely accepted on the left; there is nothing comparable to the Parekh Report's challenging of common national norms in the name of difference. Like Marshall and Beveridge, the theorists of Scandinavia's welfare states insisted on the need for national solidarity. A feeling for what she called 'patriotic pride' marked Alva Myrdal's 1941 *Family and Nation*.[14] Sweden, she happily pointed out, was a relatively uncontested idea. Its boundaries had been fixed for over 100 years. There were, moreover, no big subnationalities within its borders at the time she wrote; there were 34,000 Finns, but 'there was never any urge to enforce their total assimilation or to keep them out of the Swedish communion'.

But the days when Alva Myrdal could take Swedishness for granted are gone and the chief beneficiaries of the pro-natalist policies she advocated would no longer be poor rural or working-class women struggling to combine family and work but immigrant women who mostly do not work. While Sweden, like most European countries, invited in some guest workers during the booming 1960s and 1970s, the past two decades have seen a second wave of immigration that is unprecedented in Swedish history. According to a 1997 government report, *The Future and Diversity*, 17 per cent of all children born in Sweden have at least one foreign-born parent.[15] Within another decade, one quarter of people living in Sweden under the age of 17 will be immigrants or the children of immigrants. Similar conditions exist in Denmark. A recent White Paper, *Better Integration*, projects that by 2020 there will be 800,000 'foreigners' living in Denmark.[16] ('Foreigner' denotes immigrants and their children, including those born in Denmark.) They will then form 13.7 per cent of the population.

In both Sweden and Denmark, the second wave of immigration differs from the first, not only in numbers. Unlike the Turks and Yugoslavs who came as guest workers, the new immigrants include many Africans, Pakistanis and Iraqis. They are arriving at a time when the economy, with its tight labour market, cannot easily absorb them. New immigrants in Sweden, according to the Government, are badly educated, have poor language skills, and feel alienated and discriminated against. They also behave differently. In Denmark, where the fertility rate is 1.7 children per couple, immigrants from Somalia reproduce at a rate of 5.6 and those from Iraq at a rate of 4.5.

Priding themselves on their inclusiveness and solidarity, Sweden and Denmark give immigrants the right to vote in local elections and expend great effort thinking about how to integrate them. But these are also countries with large welfare states, in which people are used to passing on large parts of their income to strangers – until recently, strangers quite like themselves. In both languages, the term 'welfare state' is synonymous with 'welfare society', and the solidarity which underpins it is premised upon society-wide norms and a common morality.

Appeals to common moral understandings are not vague incantations. The Scandinavian welfare states assume agreement over issues which can be highly divisive in many parts of the world. In Scandinavia, for example, it is common to view gender equality as the most recent chapter in the advancing history of rights detailed by Marshall. Social policies emphasising gender equality are needed, because, without them, women cannot be full citizens, actively participating in public and private life. Support for gender equality is so deeply entrenched in these societies that the welfare state is not morally neutral between different conceptions of the family. Were the welfare state to tolerate patriarchal or authoritarian treatment of women in the name of pluralism, it would be violating the welfare state's insistence on equality.

Because the welfare state is not neutral with respect to gender equality, it also takes sides on the question of language. Immigrants are expected to learn the language of their new country as rapidly as possible: 'It is expected of foreigners who wish to live in Denmark that they will make an effort to learn Danish and adjust to Danish society,' says the *Better Integration* report. The reason is clear. Immigrant men, to the extent that they can find jobs, will join the larger society. Without command of the language, women will be unable to claim the rights offered to them by the welfare state. Hence, the state is obliged to work its way inside ethnic communities in order to ensure that everyone becomes part of the same society.

Official documents in both Sweden and Denmark insist that, for the welfare state to protect itself, immigrants must abandon any beliefs and practices that violate the norms of Scandinavian solidarity. The objective of integration, the Swedish report holds, should be 'equal rights and opportunities for all without regard to ethnic or cultural background'. Echoing Marshall's ideas about class abatement, the report argues that the purpose of policy 'should be to abate ethnic segregation'. The Danish report goes even further. 'Foreigners who are legally in the country must be introduced to Danish society in a fruitful fashion … society has to demand that foreigners act to become self-sufficient and integrated into Danish society by becoming conversant with basic Danish values. It is a truism that foreigners as well as Danes must obey the country's laws and rules.'

Compared to the Parekh Report, there is no emphasis in either document on group rights or the protection of group customs; it is individuals who have rights, not the ethnic communities themselves. Both, moreover, stress the reciprocal obligations of immigrants far more than the Parekh Report.

'The Danish welfare state faces a dilemma,' wrote law professor Stig Jørgensen, in the newspaper *Information*.[17] 'On the one hand, foreigners receive more from the state than they contribute to the common insurance pool, but on the other hand, we cannot accept different treatment between them and Danes.' The only solution seems to be to try to make foreigners more like Danes as quickly as possible. It is not enough, writes Anne Worning, the Director of the Federation of Danish Social Workers, in the same newspaper, to insist that Amra from Iran learns Danish and throws away her chador. 'If she is to become integrated as a citizen, employers have to employ her, her neighbours have to invite her in for coffee, landlords have to rent her a room, etc.' To counter the politics of exclusion proposed by right-wing parties, social democrats support a politics of inclusion. But what the Danes call integration, the Parekh Report dismisses as assimilation.

The Scandinavian insistence on solidarity and integration carries a price – as it does elsewhere in Europe. Sweden and Denmark are often viewed as among the most tolerant places in the world. Yet the defence of the welfare state in the face of the new immigration has revealed an undercurrent of racism. Also, Swedish and Danish industrial policy, which favours high-paying jobs and strong unions, exacerbates the problem by confining migrants to the margins. So, 54 per cent of men and 67 per cent of women from non-European societies are unemployed in Denmark. Since 1985, 92 per cent of Turks living in Albertslund, a Copenhagen suburb, have married other Turks. In most cases, one partner either still lived in Turkey or had arrived in Denmark that year.

For all the talk of integration, Swedes and Danes – unlike the French and Britons with their colonial pasts – have little experience of mixing with people who are different from them. The Swedish report on diversity says that 'in order for Swedish to work as a bridge between people, it is necessary to increase the tolerance Swedes have for those who do not speak the language perfectly or speak it with an accent', a formulation which suggests the existence of considerable intolerance in daily life. Integration is proclaimed but nothing like it has been achieved.

The problems that the Scandinavian countries are experiencing highlights the difficulty of clinging to the old ideal of solidarity in a globalising world with high levels of immigration. At the same time, the Parekh Report, and the many others like it, go too far in the other direction – underestimating the extent to which social solidarity requires strong national cultures. The UK seems to be navigating this divide better than many. For example, it requires all immigrants to learn English but subsidises minority languages; it imposes a common core curriculum in schools, but still allows some people to call themselves Islamic or Hindu. Attitude surveys in the UK have been recording a steady decline in racial prejudice. According to Yasmin Alibhai-Brown's book *True Colours*, 74 per cent of whites (88 per cent of young whites) said they would not mind if a close relative married an Afro-Carribean.[18] (In the hugely successful television series *Big Brother*, two of the most popular characters were a lesbian and a black man.) But there is also a significant minority who do not embrace diversity. And working-class Britons are still far more likely to hold conservative views across the range of moral and social issues, including immigration. According to the latest British Social Attitudes Survey, 60 per cent of working-class people think that sex between two adults of the same sex is wrong, which compares with only 37 per cent of the salariat. There are similar moral gulfs between the generations. The same survey records that 72 per cent of 25 to 34 year olds believe it is 'not wrong at all' if a man and woman have sex before marriage, only 32 per cent of 55 to 64 year olds agree.

What should the UK do?

The range of policy differences from the USA to the UK, to Sweden and Denmark, illustrates the challenges facing the welfare state from immigration and multiculturalism. Historically, opposition to ambitious governmental programs such as the NHS came from conservatives arguing in favour of the market or lower rates of taxation. But these days the biggest challenge to programmes rooted in the principle of social solidarity comes instead from the insistence on the part of multicultural theorists that the concept of solidarity, implying as it does the superiority of a common national culture, is insensitive to racial and ethnic difference.

The Parekh Report asks us not to allow a society's core values to turn into 'moral dogmatism' and 'unjustified cultural interference'. But at what point should society, in the name of respect for everyone's basic right to health, have to insist that core values such as liberty and dignity must be strengthened? We would claim that it is time to stake out the moral high ground when it comes to one such issue: female circumcision. Noting that female circumcision is a practice involving only some Muslims but not others, and hence does not merit protection on religious grounds, Parekh, in *Rethinking Multiculturalism*, nevertheless argues that one type of female circumcision 'involves minimum physical harm and does not seem to be very different from male circumcision'. (He supports banning other types of circumcision.) Consequently, '[a]ll that society is entitled to insist upon is that it should be done by qualified people under public supervision and medically acceptable conditions' (p.276).

Controversy continues to rage about male circumcision, but many would argue that public health providers should not even be in the business of circumcising newborn boys. Health policy experts – at least until the recent discovery that circumcision may be associated with lower HIV infection rates – have pointed to circumcision as an example of the excesses of US health care policies. We would disagree that partial clitoridectomy on pre-pubescent girls is even remotely comparable to circumcising infant boys. Leaving that aside, we also do not see how a government committed to equality between men and women can place an obligation to provide clitoridectomies upon public health care providers – even if that means that girls undergoing these procedures would have the benefit of licensed medical care.

A principle such as the fundamental equality between men and women has become a core value in the UK, as it has in the USA and Scandinavia. To be a modern Briton is to accept the idea that individuals have certain rights, including rights in their person that cannot be sacrificed merely because someone resident in the UK asserts that their particular cultural traditions demand otherwise. At the same time, conceptions of what it means to be British can, and should, change as the ethnic and racial population of the UK change. To strengthen institutions such as the NHS, so that they express both solidarity and diversity, requires a unifying idea of Britishness that can encompass diversity but is not eclipsed by it. The Parekh Report's rejection of the idea of a British way of life echoes Margaret Thatcher's famous remark that there is no such thing as society. Right-wing libertarians want business to do whatever it decides is in its best interest, irrespective of its impact on the common good, and left-wing multicultural libertarians want minorities to do whatever is in their interests, irrespective of its impact on the common good. Multiculturalists seem to believe that it is sufficient to base solidarity on abstract concepts of international law rather than real people with recognisable values and motives.

The story of modernity has been about people's ability to master forces once considered outside their control. Unwilling to grow old without some guarantee of economic security, or to face a labour market which could throw them out of work with no means of support, citizens of modern liberal democracies have pooled their exposure to risk in welfare states. In the absence of common threats, it is the shared interests we have in the effectiveness of institutions like the NHS that binds us together most. And despite the limits of social democracy, the collapse of communism, and the ascendancy of Reaganism and Thatcherism in the 1980s and 1990s, there is no mass support for a politics which would return us to the kinds of lives people led before the

20th century. Theorists of multiculturalism have rightly pointed to the vast changes in UK society since the NHS was first created. If the NHS is to function well in its new environment, however, it will do so only by insisting on one principle that has not changed: the welfare state has the right, if not the duty, to insist on ideas of national solidarity that make all other values, including the value of diversity, possible.

References

1   UK Department of Health. *Health Survey for England. The Health of Minority Ethnic Groups 1999.* (www.official-documents.co.uk/documents/doh/survey99/hse99-02.htm)

2   Marshall T H. *Citizenship and Social Class and Other Essays.* Cambridge: Cambridge University Press, 1950.

3   Beveridge W H. *Social Insurance and Allied Services.* New York: Macmillan, 1942.

4   Beveridge W H. *The Pillars of Security, and Other War-Time Essays and Addresses.* New York: Macmillan, 1943.

5   Tawney R H. *Equality.* New York: Capricorn Books, 1961 [1931].

6   Runnymede Trust. *The Future of Multi-Ethnic Britain: the Parekh Report.* London: Profile Books, 2000. References are to this Report unless otherwise stated.

7   UK Home Office. *Race Equality in Public Services.* London: 2000.

8   Parekh B. The Rushdie affair: research agenda for political philosophy. In: Kymlicka W, editor. *The Rights of Minority Cultures.* New York: Oxford University Press, 1995: 303–20.

9   Okin S M. *Is Multiculturalism Bad for Women?* Boston: Beacon Press, 1999.

10 Parekh B. *Rethinking Multiculturalism: cultural diversity and political theory.* Cambridge, MA: Harvard University Press, 2000.

11 Holmes S, Sunstein C. *The Cost of Rights: why liberty depends on taxes.* New York: Norton, 1999.

12 Shils E, Young M. The meaning of the Coronation. In: Shils E, editor. *Center and Periphery: essays in macrosociology.* Chicago: University of Chicago Press, 1975.

13 Myrdal A. *Nation and Family: the Swedish experiment in democratic family and population policy.* New York: Harper, 1941.

14 Sweden. Prop. 1997/98:16. Sverige, framtiden och mångfalden – från invandrarpolitik till integrationspolitik. (Trans.: *Sweden, the Future and Diversity. From Immigrant Policy to Integration Policy*).

15 Denmark. Bedre Integration – en samlet handlingsplan. (Trans.: *Better Integration – a Unified Action Plan.*) Rapport fra regeringens ministerudvalg vedrørende integration og utilpassede unge. (Trans.: Report from the ministerial committee on integration and felonious youth.) February 2000.

16 Dagbladet. *Information.* September 28, 1999.

17 Allibhai-Brown Y. *True Colours.* London: Institute for Public Policy Research, 1999.

Practice from the King's Fund

Chapter 13

Voices, values and health: involving the public in moral decisions

Kristina Staley

While debates over the rights and wrongs of traditional public health measures, such as banning smoking in public places, have become familiar to many, there has been much less public debate over the new public health measures - those that seek to address the social determinants of health. An urgent need to address these social factors underpins much of London's current public health policy. But there is also an accompanying need for more extensive public debate of these issues to ensure the development of policies that will receive widespread public support. This chapter discusses the main findings from a ground-breaking King's Fund project that engaged members of the public in the first debate of this kind. Londoners were asked their views on the ethical issues arising from current public health policies in London, and how they thought such controversial decisions should be made.[1]

The overall aims of the project were to:

- explore different approaches to eliciting values in a public debate
- provide a deeper understanding of what Londoners think is important in relation to public health policy
- explore Londoner's views on how public health policy decisions should be made when public values conflict.

The results demonstrate that participants were highly supportive of measures that promote collective health, and strongly believed that members of the public should be involved in public health policy decision-making. It is hoped these findings will provide a starting point for more extensive public engagement with these issues in the future.

What is public health?

Public health involves collective action by and for society as a whole. Public health policies aim to create conditions in which populations can be healthy,[2] rather than directly treating people who are ill. Traditional public health measures tackle the spread of infectious disease, for example through immunisation or provision of clean drinking water, while the new public health measures aim to tackle the social determinants of health, for example, reducing poverty and social exclusion. Strategies to achieve public health therefore include:

- preventive aspects of medical care, e.g. immunisation and screening programmes
- health education and behavioural modification, e.g. advice to give up smoking, compulsory seat-belt use
- control of the environment – physical, biological and social, e.g. measures to reduce traffic pollution, to improve food hygiene and to regenerate urban neighbourhoods.

Such strategies are usually implemented through the agencies of the state, and cannot be achieved by individuals acting alone. Debates about what ought to be done in public health therefore involve a discussion of public values and seek to define the acceptable limits on health-promoting state action. For example, should individuals be made to act against their wishes in order to promote their own health?

What is a public value?

Public values have been summarised as 'conceptions of the morally desirable in the realm of state activity'.[3] In the context of public debates, it is important to keep a clear distinction between 'public values' and the 'public's values'. The former are moral concepts; the latter are empirical findings about what position people take on those moral concepts. For example, in relation to a public health policy that aims to reduce smoking, a debate on public values would revolve around a discussion of the limits on government action to improve health through smoking cessation. It would consider normative issues such as 'would a ban on smoking in public places be acceptable?' or 'is it acceptable to place a heavy tax on cigarettes?'. In contrast, the 'public's values' are simply what the public thinks about these issues at any given point in time. In this chapter we are concerned with this empirical question, although in the course of eliciting the public's views the project took great pains to encourage the public to engage and reflect with one another on the values themselves.

But eliciting people's values is no easy task, not least because values themselves interact in complex and confusing ways. In some areas of public health policy, different public values can work in harmony – for example, policies that successfully reduce inequalities in health may also increase security by reducing risks of life-threatening disease. More often though, values come into conflict. Conflicts between autonomy and other values are the most common, since a government's desire to promote the health of the population often comes at a cost to individual freedom. These conflicts pose some of the most difficult questions for public health policy-makers and indeed for decision-makers in many other areas of public policy: How far should the state be allowed to intervene? What is the proper balance between state intervention and individual responsibility? When should people be free to make their own choices?

The King's Fund public debate

Since the pursuit of public health policy goals often involves trading-off one value against another and different people tend to trade-off values in ways that reflect their individual view of what is important, two fundamental questions are raised in relation to any public health issue:

*   what trade-offs should be made between different values?
*   who makes the final judgement?

These questions formed the basis of the King's Fund public debate. Citizens of London were asked to discuss trade-offs between values in relation to 'live' issues in the capital. They were then asked how the value conflicts should be resolved and in particular what role the public should play in the decision-making process.

The public debate itself took place in three stages: a series of discussion groups, one-day workshops and an opinion survey.[4] Since values are difficult to discuss in the abstract, participants were asked to discuss what should happen in fictional scenarios reflecting real life policy dilemmas. Their discussion of alternative practical solutions revealed what people thought and felt to be important. Two scenarios used throughout the debate are detailed in Boxes 13.1 and 13.2. In the next section, the key findings from the debate will be discussed in relation to these two issues – 'Introducing congestion charges in London' and 'Tackling inequalities in heart disease.'

Box 13.1: Issue – Introducing congestion charges in London

If there were less traffic in London, the health of Londoners would be greatly improved. The benefits for people's health include less air pollution, fewer traffic accidents, and more people using 'healthier' transport – walking, cycling, buses and the tube.

For buses to be a realistic alternative to cars, traffic needs to be reduced. At the moment, buses are unreliable and journey times are too long. Introducing congestion charges seems to be the only practical way of reducing the number of cars on the road. It would also provide extra money, badly needed for improving public transport, both buses and the tube.

Congestion charges could take the form of having to buy an extra license to drive in the central London area, a flat fee of £5 a day and/or the introduction of a workplace parking charge. The introduction of this charge could affect people in different ways.

Should the congestion charge be introduced?

Box 13.2: Issue – Tackling inequalities in heart disease

North and South Greyton have similar sized populations, but many more people suffer from heart disease in North Greyton as the population is much poorer. The number of people who die from heart attacks in the North is much greater than the national average, while the number dying in the South is just below average. The health authority and local authority plan to start a Healthy Heart campaign to encourage people to eat a more healthy diet, exercise and quit smoking. They plan to put 80 per cent of the resources into the north of the town where the problem is worse. This will enable the North to trial a new package of measures to combat heart disease, which include 'exercise on prescription', free nicotine patches, and advice from nutritionists. These will not be available in the South. This suggestion has met with great resistance at public meetings. Most people at the public meetings are from the South. Local Southern groups have got together to campaign for more resources in their area. Local people expressed their views in a phone-in poll in a local newspaper. The results were that the majority (60 per cent) thought that resources should be split between North and South 50:50.

How should the resources be divided?

Key findings from the public debate

As expected, the debate around public values proved highly contentious, messy and difficult to resolve. Different people held strongly opposing views and even individuals' own values conflicted with each other. However, some clear themes did emerge and are discussed below.

Participants' views on the issue of congestion charges

Most of the discussion on this issue revolved around the following key principles:

- whether the charges would be fair – reflecting concerns about *equity*
- whether charges would restrict people's freedom to drive – reflecting concerns about *autonomy*
- whether Londoners would support the charges – reflecting concerns about *democracy*
- whether charges would be effective, i.e. whether they would really reduce car use and deliver the potential health gains, and thus whether introducing charges is an efficient use of government time and effort – reflecting concerns about *efficiency*.

Concerns that congestion charges were inequitable and discriminated against the poor lay behind the strongest opposition to the introduction of charges. This opposition was reinforced by the conclusion that the choices of the less well-off would be more severely restricted. There were suggestions that alternative means should be sought to restrict car use that would not depend on financial status. However, none of the participants supported a complete ban on cars, indicating the limits of their tolerance for restricting individual autonomy.

Indeed, some participants opposed charges outright because they believed it to be too severe a restriction of civil liberties and an infringement of an individual's 'right to drive'. This principle of protecting autonomy gained more support from individual participants than health promotion when considered in relation to their own health. It was thought that *individuals* should be free to make choices about their own behaviour, whatever the consequences for themselves. However, when weighed against the 'health of everyone', protecting individual autonomy was perceived to be less significant. Shifting the focus from individual to population health changed participants' views on acceptable trade-offs between values. In fact, the majority of participants consistently prioritised promoting collective health and 'efficiency' over and above concerns about freedom to drive (autonomy), the fairness of charging (equity), and even popular opinion (democracy).

A large majority of the participants agreed with the statement that it is the responsibility of decision-makers to make sure our taxes are spent in the best way to improve health, even if it is unpopular. Most participants also believed that if Londoners were made more aware of the health benefits of reducing traffic they would be more supportive of the charges. In much the same way that attitudes to drink-driving laws have changed, it was thought that public opinion could be altered over time. Some participants believed that the public should be convinced of the merits of introducing charges *before* any decision was made. However, even this group (somewhat reluctantly) concluded that if the majority of people still opposed charges, decision-makers should overrule them.

Participants' views on the issue of tackling health inequalities

Most of the discussion on this issue revolved around the following key principles:

- whether an unequal distribution of resources was fair – reflecting concerns about *equity*
- whether an unequal distribution of resources would maximise health gains – reflecting concerns about *efficiency*
- whether the public would oppose an unequal distribution of resources – reflecting concerns about *democracy*.

Participants were unanimous in their support for distributing resources to ensure an equitable outcome, one in which everyone received the health care they needed. This view was reinforced by arguments for efficiency – money would be wasted if spent on a population in less need. However, participants emphasised that if resources were to be allocated according to need, then 'need' should be regularly assessed.

There was some debate as to whether it was fair for the healthier population to be asked 'to make sacrifices' for the unhealthy population. Some argued that since individuals are responsible for the decisions they make about their own lifestyle and health, the healthy population should not be penalised for 'having made good decisions'. However, participants also recognised that not all choices are 'free' and that the poorer population would require more investment to be able to make healthier choices for themselves.

Participants easily recognised that the public consultation processes outlined in the scenario, a phone-in poll and public meetings, were very likely to be dominated by people motivated by self-interest. They thought that the people who stood to 'lose out' would be more motivated to get involved and, as residents of a wealthier population, would be more politically aware and generally better prepared to 'defend their rights'. Emphasis was placed on ensuring a more rigorous system of seeking public opinion, to include those that might not otherwise be heard.

Participants were not convinced that the people who stood to 'lose out' in this scenario would ever be persuaded to act altruistically even if they understood the moral arguments for an unequal distribution of resources. They concluded that such individuals should not be given responsibility for decisions on this matter. It was thought that responsibility should lie solely with the decision-makers, who were then duty bound to act in the best interests of the population as a whole. Hence, they placed limits on the value of democracy, particularly in this context of public support for an 'immoral' decision.

Participants' views on involving the public in resolving value conflicts

Participants thought that members of the public had a right to take part in any decision-making process aiming to resolve value conflicts because they would be the people most influenced by the outcome. It was also thought that members of the public would add a 'realistic' point of view 'based on personal experience', which might otherwise be lacking. However, there was strong agreement that in order for the general public to be *involved*, they must first be *informed*. It was thought that an uninformed public would make poor decisions.

There was lengthy debate as to the limits of public involvement. While it was agreed that a wide range of views should be included, it was recognised that not all members of the public would want to be involved. Participants concluded that people should not be forced to participate against their wishes, again reflecting the high value placed on autonomy. They also emphasised that the process should be efficient. It was not thought practical to consult 'everyone on every single issue', and an additional concern was that the process should not take so long as to prohibit decisions being made. Participants argued for striking a balance between leaving decision-making to too few and including so many people that decisions could not be made quickly and effectively.

Some participants felt that the public should have the final say in resolving value conflicts. They reasoned that since a majority vote decides who should be in government, a majority vote could decide upon the actions of that government, and that only members of the public would know what was in their best interest. However, this view was opposed by those who were concerned that the public might be motivated purely by self-interest and may not be best placed to judge the effects of any decisions on society as a whole. They perceived the role of government to be to listen to the broad range of interests, not just the majority or vocal minority views, and to strike a balance between all concerns. They were therefore in favour of government having the final say, but few thought that government could make those decisions alone. The majority of participants strongly supported the view that the Government has a duty to take final decisions, but only after consulting the public and after considering as many different perspectives as possible. Participants reasoned that there was no single view that could be said to represent 'public opinion', reinforcing the need to 'embrace diversity'.

Participants recognised that it was unlikely that any public consultation would provide a single, simple answer and that all controversial decisions would inevitably be unfavourable to some. They therefore placed great emphasis on the decision-making process being open and transparent and the need for evidence of a wide range of people's views being taken into account. They thought it would be impossible to convince everyone that a decision was the 'right' one, but that the public might be more accepting of a decision if they understood the reasoning behind it. In contrast, not consulting the public at all was thought to lead to deep-felt public hostility and distrust.

In subsequent discussions on what would constitute a legitimate means of public involvement, participants spontaneously described a system similar to a deliberative model of a 'citizens' jury'.[5] This model would incorporate the features participants thought to be essential for obtaining a reliable indicator of public opinion, including time to consider information, opportunities for deliberation amongst people with diverse views and, most importantly, independence of any vested interest.

The challenges posed by involving the public in resolving value conflicts

Participants in this debate voiced strong support for involving the public in decision-making processes that aim to resolve value conflicts. Indeed, they argued that it would be impossible to involve the public in any decision-making process *without* a debate around public values. They reasoned that making any policy decision would first require a discussion about 'what ought to be done' ahead of a discussion of the practicalities of 'how to do it'.

Deliberations on the process by which members of the public might be involved in resolving value conflicts raised the now-familiar demands for:

* inclusivity: the incorporation of a wide range of views
* independence of any vested interest
* openness and transparency in the decision-making process
* greater public accountability, in particular explanation of the moral reasoning behind policy decisions.

However, this debate, as the first of its kind, was also important in highlighting the serious challenges posed by involving the public in such a process. There are clear difficulties that emerge when considering how and when the public could be involved in the decision-making. The four key challenges that came to light in this debate are now taken in turn.

Eliciting public values through public debate

In free-ranging discussions, participants did not instinctively refer to public values or matters of principle when discussing policy options. Instead, they tended either to refer to their personal experience to solve practical problems or to their self-interest in choosing between different options. They tended to explore different options only insofar as they thought these would *work*. This does not mean that values were thought to be unimportant, but does indicate that members of the public need to be encouraged to articulate their views on public values, which may otherwise go unexpressed.

In some of the group discussions, it appears that participants responded in a way they thought socially acceptable. The views they expressed in the group directly contrasted with their privately held opinions captured by anonymous questionnaire. On the one hand, this impact of the group dynamic can be viewed positively, since it would seem to promote civic-mindedness and counterbalance prejudiced opinions. On the other, there is concern that if group dynamics disguise people's true values, they could in fact hinder the progress of debate. People need to be able to air and discuss their views if their opinions are to be understood by others and, importantly, if their views are to be effectively challenged.

Resolving 'irresolvable' value conflicts

Participants recognised that value conflicts by their nature are often irresolvable and that it is impossible to satisfy all sides of a debate. However, they concluded that if members of the public could trust the process of resolving such conflicts, they might be more accepting of a final decision, even if it went against their views. But this conclusion was reached within the hypothetical discussion of fictional scenarios. Participants recognised that they might feel and act very differently in the 'real world', where a decision would have a real impact on their lives.

This issue came to the fore in discussions around tackling health inequalities and the redistribution of resources. Participants were unanimous in their support for an unequal distribution of resources in the abstract, but when they placed themselves in the position of people who would receive less, they were less accepting of the disparity. In stark contrast to the conclusions reached in relation to congestion charging, participants stated that no amount of moral reasoning was likely to convince them to accept fewer resources when that personal sacrifice was a perceived as a reduction in health care. This probably reflects people's fears for their personal security and the potential threat to life posed by inadequate health care provision.

A public debate on values cannot therefore hope to eliminate conflict or ensure public acceptance of 'morally justifiable' decisions. However, such debates could help to *limit* conflict by clarifying the exact nature of any disagreement and identifying areas where agreement might be reached.[6] In contrast, a lack of public engagement could create even greater public hostility. Processes that exclude the public are more likely to make people angry and resentful, and may further entrench individuals in their polarised positions.[7] Although deliberation of ethical issues may bring deep disagreements to the surface, it offers the chance to modify people's views through access to new opinions and new information. Such changes might help to move the debate forward.

Removing bias and ensuring representativeness when seeking public opinion

There were contradictions in participants' minds as to which members of the public should be involved in the decision-making process. On the one hand, the public were perceived as having a legitimate place at the table, because they would be the ones most affected by any decision. On the other hand, those motivated by self-interest were ruled out on the basis that they could not be trusted. It has been suggested that this dilemma could be resolved by involving the public in two capacities: first, as service users with recognised individual needs; and second, as 'disinterested' citizens with broader and longer-term interests in the fair distribution of public resources.[8] For certain types of public involvement exercise it may be desirable to *exclude* those with a particular interest, on the basis that they would not be in a position to act impartially. For example, in the case of congestion charging it might be possible to exclude those with an overt financial interest in the decision, such as public transport workers and managers.

However, it is not realistic to identify general citizens of London who do not have some interest in the policy outcome. Indeed, it has been argued that it is frequently impossible to distinguish between people who are affected by a decision and people who are not.[9] Perhaps, as some participants suggested, it is more important that the people who do participate are open and honest about their concerns to ensure that the process is not dominated by any single interest. Most importantly, the people carrying out the consultation exercise must be visibly independent of the interests of either the public or the Government.

Participants also raised concerns about representativeness and the difficulties of striking the correct balance between efficiency and democracy. They questioned how 'every voice' could be heard without making the process so unwieldy as to be impractical or prohibitively expensive. Such concerns are widely recognised, but it has also been argued that high-quality citizen input at the beginning of a decision-making process may be ultimately more efficient than low-quality citizen input, perhaps when it is too late.[10]

Balancing public and professional views – ensuring accountability and political legitimacy

This is perhaps the biggest challenge to effective public involvement. In this debate, participants' descriptions of a legitimate decision-making process involved consulting the public but ultimately giving decision-makers the final say. There is an obvious tension between members of the public not wanting to have the final say but nevertheless wanting to be listened to. How much weight is to be given to public opinion? How can those whose opinions are ultimately rejected be convinced that they have been heard?

Significant problems would emerge if the public were given full responsibility for the final decision. It would then become more important to control and constrain any possible abuse of power. Questions would be asked about the fitness of different members of the public to make decisions and the mechanisms for ensuring accountability to their community. A process that gave citizens authority in decision-making, when those people were formally accountable to no-one and able to disappear back into the community after their involvement, is unlikely to be considered politically legitimate. It is likely that 'professional' decision-makers – individuals who are continuously responsible for and accountable to the whole community – constitute an essential role in giving the whole process necessary legitimacy and authority.

However, the existence of 'professional' decision-makers creates a power imbalance that may not be possible to correct. There is a danger that those with power and authority can ensure that they are not bound by decisions reached by the public, can opt to ignore public opinion or exploit it for their own political purposes.[11] Moreover, it has been argued that the deliberative process can be so constrained as to render it 'morally and democratically irrelevant', when professional values come to dominate or divert discussions.[12] When the values of professionals and those of the public's conflict, how can we ensure that the existing power imbalances do not influence the final decision? If professionals and the organisations are to respond meaningfully and effectively to public involvement, there will need to be a radical shift in the way they and their organisations think and behave.[13]

Conclusion

Involving the public in contentious areas of public policy is likely to become an integral part of future decision-making processes; the modern populace is well-educated, wishes to be better informed and is unwilling to submit passively to the decisions of elected masters. But we should not be too dewy-eyed about the possibilities: they bring their own ethical and practical difficulties. Involving the public may, if undertaken imaginatively, make contentious decisions less confrontational; but it will not by itself resolve the difficult ethical trade-offs that are an unavoidable part of the political process.

References

1   Staley K. *Voices, Values and Health: involving the public in moral decisions*. London: King's Fund, 2001. The project was commissioned by the R&D Directorate at the London Regional Office of the NHS Executive with a view to informing the development and implementation of *London's Health Strategy*.

2 Public health has been defined by the US Institute of Medicine as 'what we as a society do collectively to ensure the conditions in which people can be healthy'. In: New B. *Public Health and Public Values: resolving value conflicts.* London: King's Fund, 2000. Download from the King's Fund web site: www.kingsfund.org.uk/publichealth.

3 New B. *A Good-Enough Service: values, trade-offs and the NHS.* London: IPPR and the King's Fund, 1999.

4 Six one-and-a-half hour discussion groups were held with 8–10 participants; two one-day workshops were held with 12–13 participants; and a total of 500 telephone interviews were carried out. All stages involved a cross-section of Londoners. Further details can be found in the project report as in endnote 1.

5 Lenaghan J, New B, Mitchell E. Setting priorities: is there a role for citizens' juries? *BMJ* 1996; 312: 1591–3; Lenaghan J. Involving the public in rationing decisions: The experience of citizens' juries. *Health Policy* 1999; 49: 45–61.

6 Gutmann A and Thompson D; see Chapter 9 in the volume.

7 Stewart J. *Further Innovation in Democratic Practice.* Birmingham: Institute of Local Government Studies, 1996.

8 Coote A, Lenaghan J. *Citizens' Juries: theory into practice.* London: IPPR, 1997.

9 Delap C. *Making Better Decisions: report of an IPPR symposium on citizens' juries and other methods of public involvement.* London: IPPR, 1998.

10 Elizabeth S. Citizens' juries: tackling the democratic deficit. *British Journal of Health Care Management* 1999; 5: 398–400.

11 Harrison S, Mort M. Which champions, which people? Public and user involvement in health care as a technology of legitimation. *Social Policy & Administration* 1998; 32: 60–70.

12 Price D. Choices without reasons: citizens' juries and policy evaluation. *Journal of Medical Ethics* 2000; 26: 272–6.

13 Pickin C, Popay J, Staley K, *et al.* Developing a model to enhance the capacity of statutory organisations to engage with lay communities. *Journal of Health Services Research and Policy* (in press).

Chapter 14

Organisational values: a case study in the NHS

Jane Keep and John McClenahan

This chapter describes how different NHS organisations have started working with staff, patients, managers and other stakeholders in order to understand values. This may involve uncovering the values that are implicit in what people in the organisation actually do, identifying the values they aspire to or making it clear that explicit values matter.

The King's Fund values programme of work examined both the *national* values of the NHS[1] and the *personal* values and beliefs expressed by Service users and staff.[2] In late 1999, this work was taken forward when the Fund joined with a range of NHS organisations to explore what happens at *organisational* level in the Health Service. This is where people have to make the connecting links between these two sets of values and live with the tensions between them.

The Organisational Values Network initially involved the King's Fund and five NHS organisations – one primary care group (PCG) and four NHS trusts. The PCG dropped out early on owing to pressures of work and an impending merger. However, a newly formed primary care trust and an additional NHS trust (the lead person having moved there from one of the original trusts in the Network, taking the values interest with her) joined later. Brief details of the Network members are shown in Box 14.1.

The Network met for the first time in January 2000 and developed a joint commitment to learn from each other's experiences, for our benefit and to help others in the NHS who might be attempting to work with organisational values. This is increasingly a subject whose time has come, because at an individual level there is something about this kind of work that engages people, and at an organisational level values are clearly important in the Health Service. Many NHS organisations are seeking to influence corporate culture, values, goals and behaviour, at least in part, in pursuit of the principles and aims set out in the *NHS Plan*.[3] Related policies from the Department of

Health, such as those seeking greater user involvement[4] and the implementation of the Government's human resources strategy[5] also have implications for organisational values and culture. It is assumed that readers of this book will agree there is merit in attempting to clarify value, meaning and purpose in organisational life in the NHS. We are not, therefore, trying to make the case that this is a worthwhile pursuit. Instead, this chapter attempts to answer the question 'what can other NHS organisations involved in values-based work learn from our experiences?'

This chapter reviews progress under three main headings:

- What are we trying to do in the Network, and how are we going about it?
- What have the Network member organisations been doing on their own account, both before and after joining the Network?
- What have we learned from our work?

The chapter ends with a section summarising our interim conclusions.

Box 14.1: Participating organisations

Organisation	Characteristics
1. Woking Primary Care Group	Home counties PCG, newly formed.
2. St George's Healthcare NHS Trust	Large south London acute hospital-based teaching trust.
3. The Royal Hospitals, Belfast	Made up of four linked hospitals on a 70-acre site – the Royal Victoria, Royal Maternity, Royal Belfast Hospital for Sick Children and the Dental Hospital.
4. South London and Maudsley NHS Trust	Large mental health trust in London, created in 1999 from the merger of several organisations including a former special health authority teaching hospital and community mental health services.
5. Wrightington, Wigan and Leigh NHS Trust	Recently merged, large acute hospital-based trust in north-west England.
6. Nelson and West Merton Primary Care Trust	Large recently formed PCT, now consulting on merging with two PCGs to form a new PCT.
7. University Hospitals Leicester NHS Trust	Very large trust formed by recent merger between three teaching hospital trusts.

What are we trying to do in the Network, and how are we going about it?

Our initial aim was to engage with a number of different NHS organisations already working on values. We would try to understand and describe what they were doing, look at the interplay between personal, professional and institutional values in practice, and explore any differences between 'espoused' or 'declared' values, and what actually happened in the organisation ('enacted' values). Initially, this process seemed fairly straightforward, but the more we attempted to work with it, the more complex it became. The project has also changed emphasis and direction several times, as we developed greater clarity about what mattered to Network participants and what was most important to achieve. This evolutionary process, with shifting goals and unexpected changes of emphasis, parallels that found during periods of change in complex systems such as the NHS.[6] We are not, therefore, at the end of this iterative process (and maybe we never will be), and so this chapter represents a report on work in progress.

What we are trying to do

Our aims and approach respond to the diversity in purpose and methods, and various levels of progress and development, in different organisations. Our working methods now also better reflect the evolving nature of this kind of work, mirrored in the organisations themselves as they have worked with values.

After several discussions it was agreed that the Network members should try to clarify some philosophical and practical frameworks for thinking, talking and doing things about organisational values. This would help with the next step of putting guiding principles into action, and also assist (via a range of methodologies) each individual organisation with its work. We wanted the Network to become a place to develop our thinking about how we work with values across boundaries and where we could discuss our anxieties about the values aspects of mergers and other structural change.

How we are going about it

The Network meets regularly to work together on what can be described as an exploratory 'journey' about values. Sometimes people who are experienced in applying a values-based approach in other contexts are invited to share their insight and some meetings now focus on individual organisations, allowing Network members to describe what they have been doing, and the current challenges they face. One member, Jane Keep, acting as a researcher, was asked to keep a record of the Network's progress, helping to make sense of any findings and describing the member organisations' initiatives.

The group has also agreed a range of operating principles. These include: a commitment to making the Network a success; observing Chatham House rules over disclosure of potentially confidential or difficult aspects of the work; recognising that Network members' values may change over the course of the project; listening attentively and respecting others' values, views and perspectives, even if we do not share them.

What have the Network member organisations been doing on their own account?

This section describes briefly what individual organisations in the Network were and are doing locally about values. The organisations have had different starting points, have been working for varying periods of time, and have a range of different focuses and approaches to their work on values. Some have sought to engender coherence around a single cluster of organisation-wide values, and others have actively fostered diversity in articulating the values of different groups and teams within their organisation. Some 'began at the top' with the board or a small group of senior managers, others have involved a wide range of people throughout the organisation from the start.

1. Woking Primary Care Group

This PCG started its work by attempting to make implicit values explicit, in order to help inform resourcing decisions in the new organisation. It undertook work on 'shared meaning' to bring together two previously different cultures. However, the PCG later withdrew from the Network, citing too many changes in its structure and working practices, and too few senior staff.

2. St George's Healthcare NHS Trust

Work on values at the Trust began at board level, following a change in both the chair and the chief executive officer. It is now led by a small core group which works with other organisational project teams on discrete values issues such as equal opportunities and diversity. An initial focus group generated a long list of values for the organisation which was summarised as six main values, and statements as to how these might be achieved. After consultation via departmental/team meetings, an action plan is intended to follow, including something similar to a staff charter focusing on rights and responsibilities. In addition, the Trust is planning to use its staff attitude survey to ask some values-based questions explicitly. Responses to the last staff attitude survey will be used as a baseline from which to measure achievement in values terms in the future. The Trust also has an ethical forum which is currently reviewing its role and remit.

3. The Royal Hospitals, Belfast

As reflected in their organisational strategic document, *Vision of Success*, values have underpinned work at the Trust for the past 14 years. These values have remained unchanged, even though the strategic plans of the Trust have changed significantly. The chief executive has been in post throughout and has consistently applied these values to the work of the board and to other work in the organisation, enabling them to be 'lived out'. The Trust has worked hard to develop union and management staff relationships as part of their values work. When faced as a board with difficult issues, they use a questioning approach which asks: 'Is this a question of principle or otherwise?' If it is a question of principle or values, they work through an ethical framework to address the issue. Disagreements are managed because conflict happens openly – with a belief that consensus is not necessary so long as the process of decision-making is fair and open.

4. South London and Maudsley NHS Trust

This Trust has a largely new management team, who have been using networking to pursue a whole systems approach to organisational development. Work started with a well-attended staff meeting where a story-telling approach was used to describe 100 defining moments that illustrate values at work. A further meeting of 167 managers was held, again using story-telling to encourage people to think about values. This was followed by away-days on the topic for both the executive group and the board. Twenty-six separate values statements were returned from departments and teams, and these were used to generate a trust-wide statement. A poster showing this central statement and all the departmental or team statements was produced, and 500 copies were distributed for continued discussion and review.

Progress on values work was assessed at a meeting attended by 120 managers where a virtues-based approach to implementing values was used. The managers were asked to vote on their top three virtues, which emerged as personal integrity, respect and friendliness. These could then form some key characteristics of management within the Trust and help to translate some of the values into behaviour.

Through the work, the management team is reflecting on the organisation's identity (post merger) and will shortly be looking at promoting a uniform set of corporate values. In addition, the Trust's local leadership development programme includes values as part of the process of development. The Trust is also exploring patient-focused approaches which will include the Trust value statement(s).

5. Wrightington, Wigan and Leigh NHS Trust

The Trust is seeking actively to engage staff in the process of articulating values. Similar work had been undertaken in one of the pre-merged trusts, in which managers teamed up with staff members and interviewed 800 staff about their working environment and lives, asking three values-related questions. People were asked to give two examples in response to each of the following questions:

- What could be done to improve your working life?
- How could you be more involved in improving services?
- How could you be more involved in your working environment?

Responses were analysed and an action plan produced, with financial backing to assist implementation of values-related changes. The newly merged Trust is now seeking to extend its work to include patients by developing a new integrated model of involvement for patients and staff.

6. Nelson and West Merton Primary Care Trust

The chief executive and new board have explored the meaning of values in the workplace and have discussed how significant they might be, but are not yet sure how these will be used in forming the new PCT. They hope to use a values-based approach to shape the culture of the new organisation, to work with managers to understand what they are doing right, and to foster developmental improvement. They hope to smooth the process of a further planned merger by developing a set of values for the new organisation. (This merger plan was awaiting the results of consultation and the Secretary of State's decision at the time of writing.) They aim to work towards a values-based culture in the new PCT, learning from past experience of mergers about what helps, and what hinders, forming a new organisation.

7. University Hospitals Leicester NHS Trust

The Trust's director of nursing moved here from Wrightington, Wigan and Leigh NHS Trust and gained board approval to start work on values. One area of her work was to help manage the cultural implications of the merger of three formerly separate acute trusts, all with very different cultures. The Trust is working on using values to play a role in developing corporate objectives and future strategic configuration.

What have we learned?

While each member of the Network will have learned different things of personal or organisational relevance, a small number of points seem of more general importance – both to Network members and potentially to other organisations working on values.

Terminology is confusing and diverse

One of the things we have found both interesting and confusing is the wide range of terminology used and assumptions made in discussions about values, and in the wider field of ethics and morals. For example, a values-based organisation is generally regarded at first glance as a good thing. Yet surely this depends both on what the values are, and how the person or group regarding the organisation from the outside thinks about the values the organisation holds or enacts. To take an admittedly extreme example, the war-time German SS could be described as a 'values-based organisation' in the sense that its members held many values in common, and often acted coherently in accordance with them, yet most people regard its values – and its actions – with horror.

In our discussions about the meaning and interpretation of values work, we have found it necessary to consider broader questions of philosophy, morality and ethics to understand more clearly what we were talking about, and how it might be better understood. Philosophers themselves acknowledge that there are no final answers, no ultimate truths. 'The most that philosophy can provide is an approach to the problem – a structured way of thinking about things, balancing conflicting arguments.'[7] So values are to some extent relative, depending on a range of factors including the personal beliefs of the person viewing or using them, and the cultural context of the time and place. Values are not static either. Their usefulness depends upon what processes were involved in articulating them in the first place, how they are used and encouraged in an organisation, and how their effects are monitored. Values come in different groupings too, for example, moral, aesthetic, intellectual, social, economic and can be seen differently – as instrumental to some larger purpose, or intrinsic and with their own identity.[8]

We have found that Network members used very different words to describe the values-based work in their organisation and they all had difficulty in explaining what they had done in ways that other people could easily understand. This was in part due to the varying concepts and vocabulary they use. NHS jargon can also stop us expressing ourselves clearly, or can mean we become unconsciously limited in the way we see the world. The problem became the subject of an animated discussion at one of the Network meetings, and helped us gain clearer insights into what each organisation was 'about' in its use of values-based approaches. Box 14.2 (right) summarises the discussion.

The Network's attempt to disentangle some of the overlapping concepts developed as follows. We have found it necessary to distinguish between ethics as a *process* of questioning how to live and act within a moral context,[9] and morality as a more *contextual* description of current social beliefs, and customs and practices of the time and place.[10] However, this distinction between morals and ethics is not often reflected in the literature, and some authors make no such distinction. Morality, then, provides a context for determining what is regarded socially as right and wrong. Much social improvement has come from the process of ethical questioning applied to (the then current) morality, challenges made to this morality, and eventually support by enough people to allow or promote change.[11] Values, then, are things held dear by the people doing the challenging, that give context and meaning to our way of being in the world, and are at least initially personal. Others may be persuaded to share similar values, by engaging in real conversations about the meaning and implications of their application.

Within moral philosophy, philosophers through the centuries have attempted to define virtues as the 'character base' of ethics and morals.[12] Sometimes they are even seen as perennial, independent of the social context of the time, or even in some sense 'of a higher order'. We found it more helpful to think of them in the context of ethics, morality and values as 'good things' or 'ways of being or behaving'.

**BOX 14.2: OUR TERMINOLOGY: WORKING TOWARDS A COMMON AND
USEFUL LANGUAGE**

Ethics   A process of questioning how to live and to act within a moral context.

Morality   Belief systems, customs and practices of the time – that provide a
context for determining right and wrong.

Values   Things that people hold dear – that contextualise our way of being in
the world. Includes things like power, money and beauty – as well as
our personal morals.

Virtues   Ways of being (in the context of ethics, morality and values).

Linked words and concepts

Ethics	Morality
Fluidity	Fixed for the time being
Conscious thought	Unconscious influence
Internal questioning (do I or we think it is right?)	Taking on board an external point of reference (do others think it is right?)
Choices about how to live and act	Sensitive to custom, practice (and organisational culture)
Challenging decisions	Being guided by the decisions of others
Matter of process	Matter of content
Locally defined	Defined by something broader than immediate and local context
The right way?	The right answer?

Participating Network members have, it turned out, some temperamental
similarities, including a preference for possibilities rather than definitive
solutions. So, we found it hard to define absolutes in values, virtues or morality
– things that are unquestionably right or wrong. For us, ideas associated with
ethics included a sense of fluidity, explicit and conscious thought, and internal
questioning about how to live and act, not the application of fixed judgements
about right and wrong. We felt it was a matter of locally defined process to
come to conclusions about the 'right' way to proceed in difficult or contentious
circumstances. By contrast, for us, morality is a more contextual concept,
embodying widespread, currently socially accepted beliefs about what
behaviours are right and wrong. Though these may change – usually slowly –

over time, this view implies that the application of ethical processes to particular situations or actions would not only take account of the personal beliefs of participants, but also of external points of reference – do other people think this is right?

Acting morally, then, would involve being sensitive to organisational culture, custom and practice. It would involve being guided by the decisions of others, as well as (perhaps sometimes even in preference to) one's own beliefs. However, it would be defined by something broader than the immediate and local context.

Values work seems to make a positive difference

Not all the organisations participating in the Network can yet report substantive progress and tangible outcomes from their work on values. However, they all believe it has an important role in the positive development of their organisation and staff, and services to patients, their families and other carers. Our researcher used a semi-structured telephone or personal interview approach to ask people in each organisation what progress had been made. The notes below are based mainly on this part of our work, in some cases supplemented by Network meeting discussions.

At St George's Healthcare NHS Trust, the work which started with the chair, chief executive officer and the board has now broadened considerably, and is having a wider impact. The organisational values are being used in such formal mechanisms as the business development framework, providing some of the criteria against which to test options. The nurse director has used the formal declaration of organisational values as a unifying theme in meetings with senior nurses across the organisation, and it now also forms part of the work of the equal opportunities group. The Trust's induction programme for new staff now starts with a welcome from the chief executive. As part of this, he introduces the organisation's declared values. Staff turnover, though reducing, is still sufficient to ensure that a substantial proportion of all staff are now aware of the importance St George's attaches to values, and all have a copy of the values statement.

At the Royal Hospitals, Belfast there has been a financial imperative to save money. Doing this in a way which retains staff commitment is never easy, but the work in the Trust on values seems to have made it less difficult. Decisions are said to be made in a values-based way – openly, informed by rational discussion and involving those to be affected. Some crucial 'symbolic' facilities for staff, such as the crèche and some sports facilities, have been retained even though financial savings could be made from cutting them back. The organisation's values have been 'lived out' by teams in the Trust, particularly in its decision-making processes, with a concern for quality and a commitment to promoting equal opportunities.

At South London and Maudsley NHS Trust, value statements have been developed and shared by both the Trust board and local teams. These have formed the basis of further work, including the ongoing development of a set of key virtues, which managers in the Trust can endeavour to demonstrate in their own behaviour.

Wrightington, Wigan and Leigh NHS Trust has undertaken considerable work towards the staff involvement initiatives from the Department of Health and NHS Executive.[13] Through this, 'the blame culture seems to have shifted, and people are using stories to describe issues and solve problems'. People in the Trust have also 'been enabled to maintain a level of calm – rather than whipping up angst or anxiety'. Members of staff in the Trust also report having learned from this work that process is as important, or sometimes even more important, than the tangible outcomes. Staff are now more willing to become involved, not just in the values process itself, but in other forms of team working across professional disciplines and departmental boundaries. One of the strong messages from the Bristol Royal Infirmary Public Inquiry is that such team working is an important cultural change needed in today's NHS.

In Nelson and West Merton Primary Care Trust, the considerable effort required to merge multiple and disparate organisations is being helped by taking into account the values of the groups involved. Making these values explicit, and comparing them with ideas from the senior management team, is allowing a more considered view of the values inherited from former constituent parts of the PCT – what should we keep and what should go?

Finally, University Hospitals Leicester NHS Trust is using a values-based approach to the development of its new organisational strategy.

Interesting – and probably unresolvable – questions remain

In our work so far we have established a number of ways of working and approaches to 'living' values, and gained considerable understanding of the complexity and diversity of the issues involved. We have reached a measure of agreement on terminology, and seen some positive impact on the services that NHS organisations provide. Through organisational story-telling, feedback and sharing of issues, we are becoming aware of the difficulties and tensions which a principled, values-based approach can help to address. However, at this stage in the Network formation, answering some of the questions we were initially faced with has raised other and more difficult questions. Many of them are deeply philosophical, and will remain unresolvable, but we continue to struggle with them.

Work on values goes to the heart of questions about organisational identity and culture. Organisational *identity* is a fluid concept in today's NHS – organisations at all levels are being restructured. Organisational *culture* is at the heart of recent approaches to quality improvements. Work on values can provide the link in redefining identity and culture in newly forming or merging organisations. We hope that by continuing to explore the following three questions – and others – we will observe further progress on enabling values to 'live' within the Network organisations.

Question 1: What is the organisation for?

Establishing or changing the culture of an organisation – expected from all NHS bodies under the Government's modernisation plan – is in essence a question of establishing, maintaining or changing its ideology and its identity. People, animals, and organisations expend great time and energy maintaining their identity, and changes which challenge this are the hardest kind to follow through.[14]

In part for that reason, mergers are hard for organisations and on the people in them, as the constituents are required to give up some or most of their previous identity. Research shows how likely mergers are to fail in their original intentions. This is mainly due to lack of proper attention to cultural issues, of which ideology, identity, established belief systems, and inculcated or enacted organisational values form a large part.[15] So the search for values is not surprisingly of potential benefit in merged or merging organisations.

This is a particularly live issue for Nelson and West Merton Primary Care Trust, which is anticipating a further merger from already merged groups of PCGs. Its managers see values as central to its future and the PCT's senior staff are starting to use the explicit articulation of values to help shape their future identity. They are also trying to understand, from their previous experiences of mergers, what happens to staff and patients – and what helps and what hinders the continued delivery of high quality and valued services during the transition. They tell us: 'We believe that values are important, and organisations are or will become better by making work on values explicit.' They think this assumption is likely to be shared by everyone working on organisational values. Wrightington, Wigan and Leigh NHS Trust is also looking to make sense of a new post-merger model for continuing to implement values which focus on staff and patient involvement.

Question 2: How far can you actively shape culture in an organisation?

South London and Maudsley NHS Trust is looking at progressing its values work with questions around how virtues-based characteristics for managers can be promoted via their leadership and management development programmes. In addition, having merged a few years ago, the Trust is reviewing its corporate identity and looking at where it is now as an organisation, and where it is heading. This will include some aspects of its values-based work – for example the board's and individual teams' statements of values. They are also faced with the issue of whether having encouraged a diverse set of value statements from different parts of the organisation, they should now have a corporate set, which could be based on the board's value statement.

Wrightington, Wigan and Leigh NHS Trust is testing its model of patient and staff involvement to see if it makes sense, whether it is focusing on the right things and how it will work in practice.

University Hospitals Leicester NHS Trust is trying to understand how far one can *push* values into larger organisations to shape culture, and how far one can *direct* the organisation this way, as opposed to enabling it to take shape. Particularly when there may be financial imperatives or post-merger organisational and process issues to consider.

Question 3: How can we tell how we are doing?

Amongst the concerns for St George's Healthcare NHS Trust at this stage is how to find tangible evidence of the benefits of values-related work. Indeed, how can one even define what would count as 'tangible'? Even with some answers to those questions, how would one establish a baseline, and assess progress against it? Would it help to be able to place values in some form of hierarchy, as for example Maslow did in relation to individuals' hierarchy of needs?[16] And what processes help in ensuring that the values articulated by the organisation become part of day-to-day practice?

The Royal Hospitals, Belfast is considering how to continue momentum in its work on values. The organisation is trying to link values into strategic planning and decision-making, particularly when faced with continued financial constraints.

In addition to these three questions, others were also raised in recent Network discussions. How do we recognise the gaps between espoused and enacted values, and what can we learn about why they exist and how they can be closed? What are the tensions between personal, professional and organisational (local/national) values, and how do people come to terms with the trade-offs they make? How can leaders and other people in organisations make sense of these issues? Which methodologies are useful in tackling challenging, complex questions like these?

Conclusions

Firm conclusions have proved hard to reach in such a complex and diverse field but we can offer some tentative ones at this stage in our work. We hope that others will find them useful as they consider the values they wish to explore, develop or use as part of their organisation's development.

First, organisations working explicitly on values are likely to have a very wide range of approaches. These will vary depending on organisational history, local context, and the beliefs of key people in the organisation, as well as their skills and knowledge around working with values. They will also vary according to the phase of the organisation's development, its interpretation of the national context and policy impetus, and local issues and challenges.

Second, work on values is complicated in part because there is no wide agreement on the meaning of terms used – either in relevant literature, or amongst those involved in the work itself. Others attempting work in this field may find it helpful, as we did, to take some time to debate and clarify for themselves what words they find appropriate to use, and how they can usefully be interpreted. Box 14.2 on page 197 summarises our ideas but others may come to different conclusions.

Third, both the organisations and the King's Fund team working in the Network have found that useful and progressive work on values can and has been done. It is too early to say with confidence how much of a positive difference this work has made to staff and patients but there are indications that it has helped in some places, some of the time.

This work takes time, resources and effort and sometimes risks finding more questions than answers. Indeed, there is at least a theoretical risk that well-meaning attempts to involve staff in articulating values, which managers then find difficult to act out in practice, could backfire. (Though we have no evidence of this happening in any of the participating organisations.)

However, we believe that explicit attention to values should help patients and staff deal with day-to-day issues such as being clearer about developing and using patient pathways, and understanding patients' needs from their point of view. It should also help staff to decide and to understand better how and why resources are allocated. Clarity about the need for trust, openness and taking personal responsibility is enhanced by explicit attention to values. Clinical governance and the need for accountability can be made clearer, and grounded in a shared understanding of *why* they matter, not just to meet managerial targets, but to make a reality of the diverse and sometimes conflicting values of multiple stakeholders. In the midst of frequent reorganisation of NHS structures, attention to more enduring values may help to provide a degree of continuity in an otherwise turbulent environment, and help keep the NHS together. The questioning will continue, but the answers will emerge only slowly.

With acknowledgements to all participating members of the NHS organisations involved in the Network for their dedication, flair, and hard work on making values real in their organisations; Steve Manning, King's Fund Health Values programme director, and Judy Taylor, project director for the King's Fund Organisational Values Network (for holding it all together), and Judy's predecessor Alison Hill (for getting the Network launched in the first place); Steve Dewar, Val Martin and other King's Fund colleagues for their work on values, and their comments on drafts of this chapter, and all the contributors to our Network meetings. To all of you, thanks.

References

1 New B. *A Good-Enough Service: values, trade-offs and the NHS*. London: IPPR and King's Fund, 1999.

2 Malby B, Pattison S. *Living Values in the NHS*. London: King's Fund, 1999.

3 Secretary of State for Health. *The NHS Plan: a plan for investment; a plan for reform*. Cm 4818-I. London: Stationery Office, 2000.

4 Department of Health. *Staff Involvement*. Health Service Circular, HSC 1999/151, 1999.

5 Department of Health. *Human Resources Performance Framework*. Health Service Circular, HSC 2000/020, 2000.

6 See, for example, Wye L, McClenahan J W. *Getting Better with Evidence*. London: King's Fund, 2000.

7 Pearson G. *Integrity in Organisations – an alternative business ethic*. London: McGraw-Hill, 1995.

8 Talbot M. *Making your Mission Statement Work: how to identify and promote the values of your organisation*. Oxford: How To Books Ltd, 2000; and MacLagan P. *Management and Morality: a developmental perspective*. London: Sage, 1998.

9 Singer P, editor. *Ethics*. Oxford: Oxford University Press, 1994: 4; and Seedhouse D. *Ethics, the Heart of Healthcare*. London: John Wiley & Sons, 1988.

10 Vesey G, Foulkes P. *Collins Dictionary of Philosophy*. London: Collins, 1990; and Petrick J A, Quinn J F. *Management Ethics: integrity at work*. London: Sage, 1997.

11 For a health example of major challenges of this kind over 150 years, see Glouberman S. *Towards a New Perspective on Health Policy*. Toronto, Canada: Renouf Publishing. Canadian Policy Research Networks, 2001.

12 For example, Pence G. Virtue theory. In: Singer P, editor. *A Companion to Ethics*. Oxford: Blackwell Publishers, 1993: 249; and Aristotle, as quoted in Rachels J. *The Elements of Moral Philosophy*. London: McGraw-Hill, 1993.

13 Department of Health, 1999 and 2000 above; and NHS Executive. *Working Together: securing a quality workforce for the NHS*. Leeds: NHS Executive, 1999.

14 Maturana H R, Varela F J. *Tree of Knowledge: biological roots of human understanding*. 2nd edition. Boston: Shambhala Publications, 1992.

15 McClenahan J W, Howard L. *Healthy Ever After: supporting staff through merger and beyond*. London: Health Education Authority, 1999.

16 Maslow A. *Motivation and Personality*. 3rd edition. New York: Harper and Row, 1933.

A combination of thinking and practice from the UK and the USA

Chapter 15

Refining and implementing the Tavistock principles for everybody in health care*

Don Berwick, Frank Davidoff,
Howard Hiatt and Richard Smith

The ethicist Will Gaylin argued that health care reform often fails because it attempts technical solutions to ethical problems.[1] Agreeing with this position, the Tavistock Group tried to develop ethical principles that might be useful to everybody involved in health care.[2,3,4,5,6] They were intended for those who are responsible for the health care system, those who work in it, and those who use it. This article describes the origins of the principles, discusses the thinking behind them, considers how they might be used, provides case studies, and reflects on where the venture might go now.

Origins of the principles

The idea that it might be useful to develop ethical principles for everybody involved in health care stemmed from the recognition that much of health care is multidisciplinary yet ethical codes usually cover only one discipline.[2] The codes may thus be used as ammunition in interdisciplinary battles rather than as tools to think about deep problems. We advanced the idea of developing ethical principles for everybody in the BMJ in 1997[2] and then convened a group to develop some principles. The Tavistock Group, a collection of people with long experience of health care and ethical debate, developed the principles, which they published in 1999.[3,4] The principles are not evidence based and have not been validated in any scientific sense. We offer them with humility as something that might be useful, but which, like any innovation, could conceivably do more harm than good.

---

*   This chapter is reprinted from an original article published by the BMJ, with only minor amendments: BMJ 2001; 323: 616–20; this is the longer version published on the BMJ web site.

We sent the first draft of the principles to many health care organisations in the USA and the UK, inviting a response. The principles were refined in response to the feedback. (The group restricted itself to those two countries, largely because of its predominantly Anglo-American membership, although people from other countries may want to become involved.)

A meeting of about 150 invited people was held in Cambridge, Massachusetts, in April 2000 to debate each principle and to consider how the principles might be used. The meeting also heard from some US institutions that had tried using the principles. After the meeting the principles were distilled further and published again.[5] As the debate has intensified and deepened, the principles have become shorter. Box 15.1 lists the seven principles.

BOX 15.1 : THE TAVISTOCK PRINCIPLES

1. *Rights* – People have a right to health and health care

2. *Balance* – Care of individual patients is central, but the health of populations is also our concern

3. *Comprehensiveness* – In addition to treating illness, we have an obligation to ease suffering, minimise disability, prevent disease and promote health

4. *Cooperation* – Health care succeeds only if we cooperate with those we serve, each other, and those in other sectors

5. *Improvement* – Improving health care is a serious and continuing responsibility

6. *Safety* – Do no harm

7. *Openness* – Being open, honest and trustworthy is vital in health care

---

The thinking behind the principles

Rights

This principle causes more difficulty than any other, particularly in the USA. What does it mean, to say that health care is a right when 40 million people in the USA and most of the world's population do not have access to health care? And isn't it even more absurd to argue that people have a right to health? The argument over rights extends back to the 18th century, with Tom Paine arguing for them and Jeremy Bentham arguing that they were 'nonsense on stilts'. For every rights holder, argued Bentham, there must be an obligation provider. But where is that provider in the case of health care or health?

Rights, he argued, are not 'in nature' but need institutions and legislation to make them real.

Immanuel Kant distinguished between 'perfect' and 'imperfect' obligations. Perfect obligations impose a duty on particular people and institutions, whereas imperfect obligations do not. In many countries health care has become a perfect obligation (for instance, in Britain, where the Government has accepted the duty to provide health care), although it remains an imperfect obligation in others. But imperfect obligations can move – perhaps through legislation – to become perfect obligations.

Amartya Sen, Nobel prize-winning economist and Master of Trinity College, Cambridge, England, explained to the meeting in April last year why it was not absurd to make health and health care a right. By making health and health care a right, he argued, we gain people's attention: a debate begins on who might have the duty to try to achieve health and health care for everybody. There is a pressure to begin implementation. And it's important also to make health a human right because the main health determinants are not health care but sanitation, nutrition, housing, social justice, employment, and the like.

Any institution adopting the Tavistock principles would be accepting the imperfect obligation to bring health and health care to everybody. That would create a tension in institutions that provide care only for those who can afford it, but the tension ought to be creative. Those working in such institutions would search for opportunities to make health and health care more broadly available, even in countries beyond their own. And there would have to be deep discomfort around actions that restricted access to health and health care.

Balance

Many of those at the April meeting wanted 'and' rather than 'but' in this principle (see Box 15.1). They hoped to escape the tension between caring for individuals and populations. Sometimes no tension exists, but often – particularly with resources – there is tension. Resources devoted to one patient will be denied to another, or they will be denied to an enterprise that might promote public health. Antibiotics might bring benefit to individuals with mild infections while harming public health by increasing microbial resistance.

This principle calls on institutions and individuals within them to think beyond individuals to populations. Yet many people's work in health care does not go beyond the care of individuals. Paul Farmer, director of the programme in infectious disease and social change at Harvard, cited the most extreme denial of this principle – the worldwide neglect of destitute sick people.

Comprehensiveness

This principle is important for understanding the continuum of health care, said William Foege, Professor of International Health at Emory University, Atlanta, Georgia. A nurse trying to help an adolescent to stop smoking is already treating a disorder, while a surgeon treating a patient with lung cancer must be both a surgeon and a counsellor. Practitioners can easily think of themselves as providing simply a technical service. We must strive to be both specialists and generalists.

Cooperation

This principle might again seem like a truism, but following the principle might lead to profound change. Even within health care there are struggles among different groups – managers and doctors, nurses and doctors – and the debate over health care, particularly in the USA, is often dominated by blame. And, despite the vogue for patient partnership, patients often feel like the recipients of care rather than partners in a process of healing.

This principle is in many ways at the heart of the Tavistock principles. It recognises that all those who work in health care depend on each other, on patients, and on those outside health care – for example, politicians, researchers and social workers. Pulling out the principle in the middle of a bitter dispute in a hospital might prove extremely useful.

Jo Ivey Boufford, Dean of the Robert F Wagner School of Public Service at New York University, argued that 'cooperation' was too weak a word. She wanted recognition that patients are 'coproducers' of health and supported the notion of 'nothing about me without me' – in other words, practitioners would not make decision about patients without their direct involvement, and health authorities would not make policy decisions without public (and professional) involvement.

Improvement

This principle means that it isn't good enough to do well. We must aspire to do better, recognising the escalating rate of new knowledge, the rapid advances in technology, that patients want to be partners, and that our health care systems are too complex, giving too much room for error and waste. Being serious about improvement (rather than simply paying lip-service) means learning the skills of improvement, being willing to accept and even encourage change, and recognising that improvement is never ending. Most health professionals have not mastered the improvement skills, and many resist change.

Maureen Bisognano, Executive Vice-president of the Institute for Healthcare Improvement, Boston, said that health care suffers simultaneously from overuse, underuse, and misuse of interventions. Problems of service and access abound. In other words, there is huge room for improvement.

Safety

The working draft of the Tavistock principles published in 1999 had only five principles.[2,3,4] This sixth one was added as a result of consultation (and the seventh was added after discussion at the April meeting). Initially there was anxiety over 'do no harm' because it is so strongly associated with doctors. But it seemed important to include because there is increasing recognition of just how much harm health care systems produce and of how policies with benign intentions can create harm.

'Do no harm', however, is impossible to achieve, pointed out Uwe Reinhardt, Professor of Political Economy at Princeton University, and John Eisenberg, Director of the Agency for Healthcare Research and Quality in the US Department of Health and Human Services. All effective interventions may harm, but the intention behind the principle is not that practitioners should never make an intervention; it is that they should struggle to maximise benefit, minimise harm and reduce error.

Openness

This last principle might be both the most banal and the most profound. Nobody could argue against being open, honest and trustworthy, and yet every day in every health care system people fail on all three counts. It's difficult to be open and honest about deficiencies in your hospital or practice. There's always a way to 'soften the blow' or 'be economical with the truth'. You worry that you might lose the trust of patients or the public, yet nothing destroys trust faster than being found to have deceived.

Experiences of using the principles

The April meeting heard from three USA institutions that had tried to use the principles. Tom Hale from the Unity Medical Group in St Louis described how they had tried using them in their outpatient setting, which covered 125,000 patients in 80 locations. They had planned to gain acceptance of the principles, integrate them into their operations, communicate them to patients, quantify and measure outcomes, benchmark their practice against the principles, and then use feedback to assess the process. In fact they became stuck with the first principle (rights): the doctors thought that profit was important and saw this as being in conflict with health care being a right. They were also worried by the abstractness of the principles and the fact that they were not evidence based. The most important change, concluded Hale, was that they were thinking about the principles.

Nancy Boucher described how the management of the Crozer-Keystone health system in the USA had found that the principles had helped them with some difficult decisions, including whether they should disenfranchise some patients to avoid a financial loss. The management worried, however, that if it adopted the principles and competitors did not, then 'the playing field would not be level'. Would competitive advantage come from adopting or not adopting the principles? A survey of staff found that they were mostly positive about the principles but worried about having the resources to implement them.

The board of Avera Health had debated the principles twice and found them 'helpful but too broad and too vague', reported Jean Reed. They did help different groups to talk together, and the board thought that they might be particularly useful when it came to decisions on forming joint ventures (you would feel more comfortable forming a joint venture with another organisation that had adopted the principles).

Validation of the principles

How might we validate the Tavistock principles? We find this a difficult question. Have the Hippocratic oath or the Ten Commandments been validated? They have perhaps been validated in that they have been widely adopted and in some countries incorporated into law. But they have not been validated in the way that new treatments or policies might be validated – through the use of randomised trials or similar methods. It might be conceivable to validate the Tavistock principles by randomly assigning them to be used in different institutions and then measure performance outcomes, including staff motivation. But such an experiment would be difficult and expensive. It seems more sensible to validate the principles by seeing if any institutions adopt them and find them useful.

Implementation

Making strategies and principles change anything is difficult. David Garvin, Professor of Business Administration at Harvard, thought that it would be important to build up a series of cases in which the principles were applied. This would make them more concrete and operational. 11 cases are described below. Some of these cases were described in the original editorial about developing principles.[2] Garvin also suggested the creation of a user's guide: a first draft is also reproduced below.

Kenneth Roth, Executive Director of Human Rights Watch, New York, considered how the Tavistock Group might learn from the successes and failures of other codes. One way to implement a code is to incorporate it into law. This is unlikely to happen with the Tavistock principles, and the US experience of trying to create a legal bill of rights for patients is not encouraging. An alternative code is an aspirational code, which assumes good faith on the part of those trying to live by it. Such codes are often formally ratified. Those who adopt the principles are expected to live by them, but there are usually no teeth. The Tavistock principles are essentially an aspirational code.

The meeting struggled with implementation, but proposals emerged and are described below. The Tavistock Group has three broad strategies: to publicise the principles and let people do with them what they will; to do more work to encourage the adoption of the principles, mainly through being opportunistic; and to try to raise money, employ some staff, and be energetic in implementing the principles. For now, the group is following the first two strategies. But we would be delighted if anybody wanted to take the lead in pursuing the third.

Appendix 1: Case studies for use with the Tavistock principles

One test of the value of a set of principles is whether they prove useful in discussing, understanding, and deciding what to do in individual cases. Descriptions of using the principles to think about cases should allow a deeper, more operational definition of the principles. The descriptions should also be useful for education.

We begin here by using the principles to elucidate the cases we described in the original editorial (plus two others) that argued the need for principles that would apply to everybody in health care. All of these cases were based on real cases. We hope to build a bank of cases. Please send us cases, preferably with an account of how you have used the principles to think about them and whether they helped you to decide what to do.

Case 1: Denying patients a new treatment

A doctor working in an NHS trust thinks it wrong that his patients will be denied a new treatment for cancer (the hospital formulary committee had decided that it should not be prescribed). Should he contact the local media? Should the trust punish him if he does?

The 'balance' principle recognises that a tension exists between what is good for individuals and for populations. It was probably on these grounds that the committee decided that the new drug would not be made available. The 'cooperation' principle suggests that the doctor should cooperate with his colleagues and implies that contacting the media would not be helpful. But the 'openness' principle means that the committee should be open with patients, doctors and the community (through the media perhaps) on why it is denying patients a drug. The doctor might decide that the hospital is not living by the openness principle and so contact the media himself. If he does that, he should abide by the openness principle and give the whole story, not just his version. If the trust has lived by the principles and the doctor has not, then it might be legitimate to punish him. It clearly would not be legitimate if the doctor lived by the principles but the trust did not.

Case 2: Whether to share a new treatment

A staff surgeon employed full time by a 'not for profit' US health maintenance organisation develops an approach to post-operative pain control for a surgical procedure that shortens average length of stay by 1.5 days. Is she ethically obliged to share information of her discovery with the world?

Six principles (rights, balance, comprehensiveness, cooperation, improvement and openness) suggest strongly that she is obliged to share the information. The clause in the cooperation principle that says that health care succeeds only if we cooperate with 'each other' implies a loyalty to the organisation that employs us, which might be interpreted as meaning that she should not share the information. But the broader obligations in the cooperation principle – to those we serve (perhaps patients everywhere), each other (which must include many beyond our organisation), and those in other sectors – means that the information should be shared. The principles suggest that the information should be shared.

Case 3: Putting your patient before the community

A British general practice that plans to become a fundholding practice deliberately keeps its prescribing costs high for a year so that it will receive a bigger budget in its first year as a fundholder (the budget is based on the previous year's activity). Is this defrauding other practices and health organisations or doing the best for the patients in the practice? (NB Fundholding has disappeared from general practice, but the principle lives on.)

The case involves dishonesty and untrustworthiness and so is a clear breach of the 'openness' principle. Three principles (rights, balance and comprehensiveness) recognise the commitment to the broader community, which is breached in this case. The practice would also be breaching the 'improvement' principle ('improvement' means not only clinical but also organisational and economic improvement). The 'safety' principle may also be flouted because the prescribing seems to be unnecessary and every prescription carries the possibility of harm. Use of the principles suggests it would be wrong deliberately to keep prescribing costs high.

Case 4: Are the costs of improvement excessive?

> *A health maintenance organisation in the USA considers investing in improvements in its system for caring for patients with AIDS. The vice-president for marketing warns that such improvements may lead to selective enrolment of unprofitable members – namely, those with HIV infection. Is the organisation ethically bound to improve its HIV care, even if that may reduce its financial viability?*

The 'improvement' principle states that improvement is a serious and continuing responsibility. The 'balance' principle recognises the tension that may exist between the needs of individual patients and those of the population, and this principle should be considered if the investment might threaten services to other patients. The 'safety' principle suggests that it would be wrong to retain a deficient system because avoidable harm could result. The 'rights' principle means that it would be poor behaviour to seek to deny the right to health care by avoiding changes that might attract more patients. According to the principles, it would be wrong not to make the investment.

Case 5: More private beds in a public hospital

> *An NHS trust hospital wants to open more private beds to generate income to underwrite other activities. Patients entering these beds will be treated more quickly than those entering NHS beds. How do the doctors and managers square this with a commitment to put clinical need first?*

This proposal does not seem to breach any of the principles, meaning that the principles do not say anything on equity. Some argued at the meeting in Cambridge in April 2000 that they should. The 'openness' principle means that the managers would have to be open about what they were doing, which would include being open about the fact that they seemed to have breached their own 'commitment to put clinical need first'. They would need to explain why. The principles suggest that opening the beds would be acceptable so long as it was done openly.

Case 6: Withholding confidential information that could allow improvement

Newly published 'league tables' (or 'report cards') on health care providers in a region show extraordinarily good surgical outcomes in some facilities and much worse outcomes in others. The source data are held to be confidential by the auditing organisation. A hospital with poor outcomes requests information so that it can learn from high performers. Who, if anyone, is obliged to share that information? What if the performance difference is not in surgical outcomes but in waiting time?

All seven principles suggest that it would be right to share the information, no matter whether it was to do with surgical outcomes or waiting lists. If promises have been made to patients about the confidentiality of the information, then the 'openness' principle would mean that that information could not be shared without going back to the patients for consent. If the concern is around commercial secrecy, then parts of the 'cooperation' principle and 'openness' principle might be important – but it's hard to see that the concerns would outweigh all seven principles, suggesting that it would be the right thing to share the information. The principles suggest that the information should be shared.

Case 7: A nurse with HIV infection

Managers of a health provider discover that one of their nurses is infected with HIV but has told nobody. Should they release the nurse's name to the media? Should they notify all those who may have been treated by the nurse even though the chances of anybody being infected are vanishingly small?

Four principles (balance, comprehensiveness, safety and openness) suggest that the media and patients should be fully informed. The 'cooperation' principle may be taken to mean that the nurse's name should not be released without her consent. If the nurse did not consent, judgement would have to be made about releasing the name, but the weight of the principles suggests it should be disclosed. The principles favour disclosure.

Case 8: Priority setting

Should a health authority offer a new expensive treatment for Alzheimer's disease to all patients, even though it will mean diverting funds from elsewhere, including support for carers of patients with Alzheimer's disease?

Two principles (balance and comprehensiveness) recognise that the health authority is right to consider the balance and not to jump immediately one way or another. Two principles (cooperation and openness) mean that the health authorities should be open about the decision and include all parties, including patients (where possible) and carers. Two principles (improvement and safety) may be helpful in emphasising the duties to improve and to avoid harm. The principles cannot be used to make the decision, but they give strong guidance on how to make the decision.

Case 9: Selective enrolment of patients

A managed care organisation targets its marketing selectively to enrol healthy people and to avoid or discourage vulnerable populations. Is this marketing behaviour ethical? Does the answer depend on whether the organisation is owned by stockholders or is a 'not for profit' organisation?

Five principles (rights, balance, comprehensiveness, cooperation and openness) point to selective enrolment being wrong. The 'cooperation' principle recognises that employees have an obligation to owners, which in some cases includes the right to make a profit. But the principles point strongly to selective enrolment being unethical.

Case 10: Sedating an awkward patient

A doctor and a nurse decide to sedate an awkward demented patient by slipping a sedative into his tea. The nurse is afterwards disciplined. The doctor is not.

It is hard to see any justification for sedating a patient for 'a quiet life', and the doctor and nurse presumably sedated the patient because they judged the patient to be a danger to himself or others. The alternatives might have been restraint or isolation. Four principles (rights, cooperation, safety and openness) suggest that to drug the patient would be wrong, but they would also weigh against restraint or isolation. The 'balance' principle suggests that some 'harm' to the patient might be acceptable for a 'benefit' both to the patient and the population. The principles suggest that the sedation may be inappropriate. They certainly support very careful recording of all ethical considerations before action is taken. The cooperation principle suggests that it makes no sense to treat the nurse and the doctor differently.

Case 11: Denying cardiac surgery to children with Down's syndrome

A hospital with limited resources and long waiting lists was less likely to offer cardiac surgery to children with Down's syndrome.

The 'balance' principle recognises that the needs of individuals and populations must be balanced, but the 'rights' principle means that all people, no matter whether they have Down's syndrome, have a right to health care, including cardiac surgery. The 'openness' principle means that such a policy could be possible only if widely debated, including beyond surgeons and the hospital. The principles do not immediately rule out such a policy, but they do make clear that wide debate would be needed.

Appendix 2: The Tavistock principles: a user's guide

- Create an information pack that includes the principles, articles that describe how they came about, the thinking behind them, and a collection of cases. All of the material can be reproduced free without any need to contact the publishers.
- Understand that the principles are not cast in stone and can be used in any way that you want. Similarly you can adapt the background material in any way you want and add your own material.
- Find a champion to encourage use of the principles. Form a small team – preferably multidisciplinary and with a consumer/patient representative – to steer the process.
- Decide what you hope to achieve through use of the principles. It might be:
  - (a) A raised consciousness of the ethical issues of health care
  - (b) Better or different conversations about the issues that the management and practitioners face every day
  - (c) Routine use of the principles by management or practitioners

    (d) Changed behaviours; define how these will be different

    (e) Better outcomes for individuals, communities or the organisation: be specific.

- Develop a plan for achieving your aims. This might include:

    (a) Disseminating the principles and the package of information

    (b) Encouraging the senior management to adopt the principles

    (c) Encouraging (or even requiring) everybody in the organisation to adopt the principles

    (d) Publicising the principles in the community you serve

    (e) Involving consumers/patients in the process

    (f) Educational sessions

    (g) Discussions by management, teams or individuals on using the principles in everyday activities

    (h) Asking consumers/patients about whether the principles are being 'lived'

    (i) Developing measures on the use of the plan

    (j) Feeding back on what patients/consumers think and whether agreed measures are being reached.

- Implement the plan, review regularly, feedback, revise the plan as necessary.
- Share your successes and failures with others trying to implement the principles.

Appendix 3: Possibilities for implementing the Tavistock principles

- Rewrite the principles and publicise them. *This has happened.*
- Create a web site that would include the principles, background material, a user's guide and case studies. *Not done, although this article by Berwick et al. (and the accompanying material on the bmj.com) is a beginning.*
- Establish links with national and local organisations that might want to adopt and promote the principles or share experiences with those who are already adopting these or similar principles. *The American Hospital Association and the King's Fund in London are interested in promoting the use of the principles. The Partners Care Group in Boston, Massachusetts, is experimenting with the principles, and its project leader, George Thibault, can be contacted at GThibault@partners.org.*
- Encourage the use of the principles in educational institutions. *No progress.*
- Seek more involvement with consumers. *Little progress, although we are hoping to publish articles on the principles in US and British newspapers.*

- Organise a follow up meeting. *This was planned for London in spring 2002.*

References

1   Gaylin W. Faulty diagnosis. Why Clinton's health-care plan won't cure what ails us. *Harpers* 1993; October: 57–64.
2   Berwick D, Hiatt H, Janeway P, Smith R. An ethical code for everybody in health care. *BMJ* 1997; 315: 1633–4.
3   Smith R, Hiatt H, Berwick D. A shared statement of ethical principles for those who shape and give health care: a working draft from the Tavistock Group. *Ann Intern Med* 1999; 130: 143–7.
4   Smith R, Hiatt H, Berwick D. Shared ethical principles for everybody in health care. *Nursing Standard* 1999; 13 (19): 32–3.
5   Smith R, Hiatt H, Berwick D. Shared ethical principles for everybody in health care: a working draft from the Tavistock Group. *BMJ* 1999; 318: 248–51.
6   Davidoff F. Changing the subject: ethical principles for everyone in health care. *Ann Intern Med* 2000; 133: 386–9.

Commentary

The Tavistock principles: something more than rhetoric?

Alan Williams

As I have observed elsewhere:[1]

> Ethical discourse is typically inconclusive. There are good reasons why this should be so. The premisses on which it is based are usually contestable. There is usually more than one principle in play. No single principle 'trumps' all others. The situations that are selected for analysis are complex ones where the appropriate resolution of the ethical difficulties is not self-evident ...

> Helping people to be clear in their own minds about the ethical implications of their actions is not a trivial pursuit, and in the context of publicly accountable decision-making it is especially important, since the principal actors are expected to be able to provide justification for their actions, and not to behave arbitrarily or capriciously. But it is not sufficient for them merely to list the various things they claim to have taken into account. The citizenry are entitled to know what weight they gave to each, so that they can see what it was that proved decisive. Otherwise the same bland listing of relevant principles could provide justification for almost any decision.

The Tavistock principles are a good example of what I had in mind when I wrote those words. Moreover, working my way through the 11 case studies offered as examples on which to practice one's skills as an ethicist, simply bore out my final observation, because wherever a definite recommendation was made by the expert panel, I could have justified a different recommendation without stepping outside (my interpretation of) the principles on offer.

It could of course be argued that this is fine, because this is what the promoters of the principles want people to do, and so long as they can come up with a justification and are prepared to defend it publicly, their purpose will have been served. The implication of this is that the general citizenry out there are to be regarded as some kind of jury, that will ultimately determine which decisions are ethically acceptable and which are not. And from this we shall eventually distil some kind of case law about which principles are to be adduced, and given what weight, in which context. This populist stance is fine by me, though I am not at all clear how such a jury system is going to work. I suspect that the public exposure of difficult decisions with their associated ethical arguments (pro and con) might well get transmogrified into trial by media coverage rather than trial by 12 good citizens and true. It will nevertheless be a good test of the willingness of the professionals to expose their judgements to public scrutiny, and for that alone I would support it.

As regards the principles themselves, I have some deep reservations. The deepest concerns the terminology of 'rights'. 'Health for all by the year 2000' was such a right, trumpeted loudly by the World Health Organisation until it was realised what vacuous unattainable nonsense it was. The first Tavistock principle is even more vague, claiming there to be a right to health but without offering a date or timetable for its attainment (still less a definition of health that would enable us to measure progress towards its attainment). What does this 'right' mean? Does it mean that everyone has a right to perfect functioning for the longest lifespan that anyone has ever achieved? Or is it a more circumscribed 'right', for instance a right not to be more than 10 per cent worse off (somehow measured) in health terms than the average for the community in which you live? What redress do you have, against whom, if this 'right' has obviously been denied you? Can you claim redress from the International Court of Human Rights, and who is going to pay up? It seems to me still to be the same empty rhetoric as 'Health for all by the year 2000'.

The 'right to health care' is more meaningful than the 'right to health', but it cannot be an unqualified right. Archie Cochrane campaigned in the 1930s for 'all effective health care treatments to be free', a slogan which I have supported in a somewhat modified form as 'all cost-effective treatments should be free'.[2] But this is a severely circumscribed 'right', which can be made more or less attainable according to where you set the cost-effectiveness threshold. Nevertheless, circumscribed though it is, it rests on some quite important ethical principles about whether a health gain is to be regarded as of equal social value no matter who gets it, or whether the young should have priority over the old, and so on. But it poses these issues in a context in which they have to be settled specifically and quantitatively rather than by appeal in qualititative terms to vague generalities.

And why, in the second principle, is the individual patient 'central' and the whole population merely an 'also ran'! Should not the position be reversed? A *national* health service is not the same as a *private* health service. A private health service makes its own particular patients central, and everyone else 'also rans'. But a national health service should be making the whole population central, and trying to ensure that it is the appropriate people who turn up as patients. Once they are there, of course, there is a duty to offer them the same (cost-effective) treatments as would be offered to any other member of the population in their particular circumstances, but it is the decision about entitlement that is central. What I want clinicians primarily to explain is why their policies are what they are. As a secondary consideration I might later want to know why they seem to have treated Mrs X in a different way from others like her, but my primary concern is population-based.

I also think it is strange that principle 5 concentrates on the duty to improve health care, when I would have thought that the primary duty is to improve health. It might be argued that this latter concern is covered by principle 1, but if so we surely do not need principle 5, because as a consequence of principle 1 it will be necessary to improve health care (i.e. to make it more cost-effective), unless what is envisaged in principle 5 is improving the welfare of those who work in health care. And if principle 1 means doing whatever is necessary to improve the health of the population as much as possible, we surely don't need principle 6 either, since it simply says don't do anything that seems more likely to worsen people's health than to improve it!

So in my view both the substance and the language of these principles are faulty. I would find it more attractive to talk about the relative strength of different moral claims and duties in specific situations, related to the broad objectives of a national health care system (which might differ from one system to another, and over time for any one system). Why not start from a statement about the assumed objectives of the health care system (e.g. to improve the health of the whole population, and to reduce inequalities in health within that population) and then go on to identify the ethical issues that have to be confronted when pursuing those objectives? These ethical issues should then be transformed into moral constraints and duties, graded according to the weight they should have when any conflict occurs. To give but one example of such a moral constraint, to which I would attach a lot of weight, I think that only in the most exceptional circumstances should anything be done to an individual without his or her informed consent. Although I do not think that an individual has a 'right' to 'demand' health care when the generally applied and approved policy is that someone in their circumstances should not be offered it, I do think that people have the 'right' to refuse any treatment that is offered, and they should know that they have that 'right'.[3]

Let me end on a note of agreement with the authors of the principles. I think there are grave dangers in two unthinking positions that some people adopt. The first is that there are technical solutions to policy problems which are so self-evidently good that ethical argument is irrelevant. It never is. The second is that ethical argument will lead you to *the* right conclusion. It won't. There is likely to be more than one 'right' conclusion, if by 'right' you mean one that can be supported by a respectable ethical argument. In the field of ethics everything is contestable! But that does not necessarily mean that ethical argument is useless. What it can do is help reveal what it is that the ethical commentator attaches greatest weight to, compared with what you attach the greatest weight to. That is what is happening here between me and the authors of the Tavistock principles. But if it is the weights attached to rival positions by the general citizenry that are to be decisive, perhaps there is a role for rather more careful population-based research on the public's views about the relative strength of the different moral claims and duties of the various participants in the health care system. But any such research needs to go beyond developing a list of attitudes and their respective gradings, and get to the point where it is possible to elicit the actual trade-offs that people would be willing to make at the margin between the various desiderata (i.e. how much of one they would sacrifice to get a bit more of another). Until we get some rough idea of the magnitudes of the sacrifices (in overall population health, for instance) that people are willing to make in order to satisfy other desiderata, I am afraid that the professionals will be left to do the best they can with very little guidance and support from those they purport to serve.

References

1 Williams A. How economics could extend the scope of ethical discourse. *Journal of Medical Ethics* 2001; 27: 251–5.
2 Williams A. All cost-effective treatments should be free … or how Archie Cochrane changed my life! *Journal of Epidemiology and Community Health* 1997; 51: 116–20.
3 Anyone who has ever tried to discharge him/herself from hospital will appreciate the importance of this 'right' and the difficulties involved in exercising it!

Endword

Julia Neuberger and Bill New

The values debate will continue. The question that remains is whether any of the constructive proposals for developing community-owned discussions of trade-offs can be taken forward. The political mood is schizophrenic. On the one hand, the Government appears to be moving to ever more central control of the NHS. On the other, it argues that control will move nearer the patients, with the implication that Service users will be asked to participate in the discussions about what to value dear, and what not.

If bringing the NHS closer to the patients is to mean anything, then they must be allowed to enter into the debate and to decide which services they most want and how they want them provided. No-one expects the NHS to be able to do everything for everybody, but this volume demonstrates that decision-making that is value-driven may take longer, and be more deliberative, than decision by instruction from on high, but it is likely to have far greater ownership.

If the NHS is the public service most valued by most people in the UK, then wide ownership of its decision-making is critical. The values that drive its decision-making need wide dissemination. The people who use the Service deserve widespread respect.

This will not be an easy agenda. But this volume demonstrates the level of interest, and the capacity for involvement of a wide range of people. They deserve to be heard, and this book makes it clear that they would welcome being heard, in conjunction with the academic community, shaping the decisions and engaging in the trade-offs necessary in any public health care system.